BEYOND CHAOS

One Man's Journey Alongside
His Chronically Ill Wife

BY GREGG PIBURN

ARTHRITIS
FOUNDATION®

PUBLISHED BY
THE ARTHRITIS FOUNDATION

Piburn, Gregg.
   Beyond chaos : one man's journey alongside his chronically ill
wife / by Gregg Piburn.
      p. cm.
   ISBN 0-912423-20-X (pbk.)
   1. Chronically ill—Family relationships. I. Title.
RC108.P53 1999
362.1'96044' 092–dc21
   [B]   98-31883
                                                                  CIP

Published by
Arthritis Foundation
1330 West Peachtree Street
Atlanta, GA 30309

Printed in the United States of America
First printing 1999

ISBN: 0-912423-20-X

Editorial Director: Elizabeth Axtell
Art Director: Audrey Graham
Production Director: Elizabeth Compton
Interior Production: Jill Dible

Special thanks to the following individuals for their help with this project:
Janet Austin, PhD; Teresa Brady, PhD; Doyt Conn, MD; Sara Horton; Alicia
Johanneson; Cindy McDaniel; Bill Otto; John Winfield, MD.

TABLE OF CONTENTS

SECTION FOUR: FIGHTING BACK, IN THE LIGHT . .

PROLOGUE

THE BOOK
& ITS AUTHOR

(The rest of the book will be far
more meaningful and helpful if
you take a few minutes to read the
six elements of the prologue.)

Introduction

— *or* —

"Breaking the Rules"

My buddy John and I were driving a company Taurus on a two-lane road through the Colorado prairie. We were returning from a corporate speaking engagement and our conversation turned to personal issues, as they always did when we spent time together.

"Gregg, how does it make you feel to have Sherrie sick for so long?" John asked. Unlike other friends and acquaintances, John was not afraid to dig deep into my psyche, which felt abused by my wife's chronic conditions.

"Well, I certainly feel sad, especially for Sherrie," I answered. "But, you know, I'm sad for the kids and me, too." The car's speedometer read 60 mph.

"You're thinking too much," John said, jabbing my shoulder with his fist, which was the size of a linebacker's. "What does your heart say?"

I began to understand how people feel when Mike Wallace interviews them. "OK," I said, "I'm mad – mainly at her conditions." 65 mph.

"What about her operations?" I squeezed the steering wheel and remained silent. "C'mon," John pleaded, "don't clam up on me now!" Bingo!

"Yeah, I've got feelings," I screamed. "Like when I think of hospitals, I get scared. After every one of the operations Sherrie looked dead or close to dying. She always has white lips, her hair is matted, and her speech is slurred. She wears her pain on her face. White-smocked doctors walking around like they were gods, cutting open my wife and sewing her back up, making the obligatory summary speech to me in the waiting room, always saying things went great, acting as if they had swooped down from heaven to save the damn day." 75 mph.

"At least Sherrie slept through much of that crap. I'm the good little boy who had to sit in those putrid waiting rooms with my little laptop computer so I could write how wonderful it would be when the royal doctors would get done and everything would be like the old days. Pecka pecka pecka peck peck."

John said, "Now we're getting somewhere. What has it really been like?"

"For years nobody asked me that question! Everybody wants to know how Sherrie is, but what about me? We were always going to be so independent. For months we had people bringing meals, sending cards, watching the kids, scrubbing toilets. I thanked them for doing it, but hated them having to. Then they wanted to give me money. I didn't need their damn money! I needed Sherrie to get well and I needed to let my own guard down – always acting so cool, so in control, so strong. I . . . am . . . just . . . plain . . . pissed!"

We topped out at 90 mph and silence filled the car. Then I took a deep breath – the breath of a prisoner set free.

That prairie drive proved rough and wild in many ways. John and I broke some "rules," which forced me to dig deep into the river of truth. Most friends refuse to do that. I broke the rules most support people or caregivers live by when dealing with chronic illness. I tapped into my emotions and found an underground gusher. And for a man balancing way too many responsibilities and worries on my shoulders, even exceeding the speed limit felt medicinal. I am thankful we broke all of those "rules" that fall day in 1989.

Who Should Read This Book?

Nearly half the U.S. population has some form of chronic illness, such as diabetes, arthritis or ulcers, according to an item published in the *Journal of the American Medical Association*. This book is primarily for those physically healthy people who love those millions of people who feel sick day after day, year after year. But I have found through my previous writing and speaking, that people who are sick also find insight in what I have to say about my failures and successes coping with my wife's illness. You will get the most out of *Beyond Chaos* when both the support person and the ill person he or she loves read and discuss its insights together.

The Slant

Let me be clear about something from the start. In no way do I belittle in this book the challenges of people who deal with the physical aspects of chronic illness first hand. Instead, I believe I point out the difficulties of living with a chronically ill loved one, even though I know my path has been easier to travel than Sherrie's path, since she must also contend with physical ailments.

I also do not make myself out to be a "victim." Too many individuals and groups already crowd the victim rolls. While not portraying others or myself in that light, I do want readers to better understand the challenges and complexities of being affected by illness while personally being physically healthy. The purpose of this book is not an attempt to put myself on a pedestal either. Much of it reveals the mistakes I made, often making me come across as a creep. I expect some readers to dislike my behavior, and me, at certain points along my journey's path. That's fine, as long as they take something worthwhile from my words and actions.

While *Beyond Chaos* does not refer to cases in which children are chronically ill, many of the themes and suggestions noted will help those families as well. Your passage through the book will be rough and wild at times, depending on the emotional depths to which you dare to travel.

Doctors, psychologists or people who are sick write most books about chronic illness. I'm none of those. This book travels off the beaten path because a physically healthy person whose wife is sick writes his thoughts and feelings. Support people typically squelch their feelings and voices. My impetus for writing *Beyond Chaos* was to take a detour from the road traveled by other authors of books of this genre and expose the rarely voiced thoughts and feelings of someone who provides support for people diagnosed with a chronic illness. Where others whisper, this book shouts. And just when you get used to the clamor, the book whispers.

The Book Format

Beyond Chaos consists of four sections, each having three chapters. Each chapter presents a series of easy-to-read essays. The four sections in which the book has been divided relate to a group-dynamics philosophy called "The Four Phases," which describes how individuals and groups communicate and work together as they create relationships. The wide-ranging essays follow a natural progression that illustrates moving from phase one – pseudo-community – to phase four – community – in conjunction with the way I related to my wife and her illness. (See Page 13 for a brief description of "The Four Phases.")

Essay topics range from hugs to threats, from guilt to confidence, from China dolls to masturbation, from love to emotional affairs, from connections to addictions, from truth to lies, and from grief to growth. By writing about my experiences and insights, this book gives voice to millions of people who cope with a loved one's illness.

I end each section with an action page to encourage personal reflection and possible action by the reader. These pages allow you to think through the insights and experiences noted in each chapter of that section and determine how you might apply them to your situation.

Driving Forces

The day after Frank Sinatra's death on May 14, 1998, a critic noted that the famous entertainer's key to success was "singing with his guard down." I have tried to write this book with my guard down, which is the opposite behavior of many support people. Ken Burns produced the highly acclaimed documentaries "The Civil War" and "Baseball." His artistic credo is this: "If it has no emotion, it has no meaning." In other words, sharing emotions is a powerful way to "turn on more lights" of understanding. I am starting to make Burn's statement my relational and communication credo as well. People who love and support the chronically ill often believe they must be solid rocks, silently shouldering the burdens brought on by chronic illness. That strategy figuratively "turns off the lights," forcing couples and families to battle chronic illness in darkness. A lack of communication also nearly broke my relationship with Sherrie, so now I speak and write from the heart as well as the head.

The great American writer E.B. White wrote, "People like to read about a man rather than mankind." Please excuse the gender bias in Mr. White's statement. I believe he was saying that humans appreciate stories about other humans. By reading the following pages you have the unique opportunity to peer into the minds and hearts of real people who share some of the same challenges you face. You won't find a fairy tale ending, but I believe you will find some nuggets of knowledge to help you deal with your unique circumstances.

The great Swiss psychiatrist Carl Jung wrote, "If you have nothing at all to create, then perhaps you should create yourself." Writing this book is one way I chose to recreate myself and take back some of the control I lost when chronic illness ambushed my wife. My goal is for the book to help readers recreate themselves and their relationships while battling chronic illness or "The Intruder," as I have come to call Sherrie's condition.

Summary
This book does NOT:
- Belittle chronic illness and people challenged with it.
- Provide medical diagnoses or remedies.
- Focus on a particular illness.

- Follow a typical self-help book format.
- Offer simple solutions and a fairy tale ending.

This book does however:
- Encourage readers to become open, honest and courageous.
- Focus on the impact of chronic illness on those who love and support a chronically ill person.
- Delve into the emotional realm of dealing with the illness and its ramifications.
- Reveal how to progress toward a more healthy way of relating to one another.
- Offer insight and a sense of hope.

A Note About Sherrie

— *or* —

The Catalyst for the Book

Even though this book is not primarily about Sherrie or her illness, it developed as a result of her health problems. Knowing about Sherrie's health problems will help you put my thoughts and feelings into context. So here's a brief rundown of her medical history.

In 1985, when Sherrie was 31 years old, she came down with some flu-like symptoms – exhaustion, muscle pain and migraine headaches – in addition to depression. We expected the symptoms to go away within hours or days. But, of course, they did not. Her illness baffled doctors for six months before one finally told us she probably had one of the forms of Chronic Fatigue Syndrome (CFS). In 1990, some doctors finally determined that she had fibromyalgia, a musculoskeletal disorder that affects the muscles and muscle/bone connections. Her fibromyalgia symptoms have fluctuated throughout the years, but have never vanished.

Because of being diagnosed with fibromyalgia, Sherrie was forced to quit her wellness career, which included teaching aerobics, cross-country skiing and racquet ball. To complicate matters, she also underwent two major gynecological surgeries and three spine surgeries between 1986 and 1995, none related to fibromyalgia. Here's a quick rundown of her surgeries:

- An oopherectomy (removal of an ovary) in 1986
- A hysterectomy in 1987
- A laminectomy (back surgery) in 1988
- A lower-back fusion in 1989
- A neck fusion in 1995 (*Note*: I'll take the blame for this one. I hydroplaned off Interstate 25 near Denver one day and the van I was driving ended up on its side at the bottom of a ditch. Our three children and I were unharmed, but the accident created neck problems for Sherrie.)

In 1996, Sherrie's health improved dramatically. She played a key role in a community theater production, performed as a paid "extra" for two days of filming for a TV movie, and occasionally sang solos at church. But yet again, the plot of her life took a negative twist. In December of that same year, while driving to a voice lesson in a nearby town, a semi-truck turned in front of Sherrie's immobile van and clipped the front fender. As of this writing, Sherrie is trying to overcome hip and lower-back pain caused by that accident. Another surgery – to deal with this latest problem – might be necessary.

What does Sherrie think of this book? In May 1996 she gave me her blessing to focus my time and effort on writing it. I appreciate the courage it took for her to read through the essays, many of which brought back horrid memories, and offer suggestions. Sherrie asks one favor of readers: Please do not contact her with questions about her illness or advice on potential cures. She has an excellent medical team in place and would prefer not to be contacted by outsiders.

I considered Sherrie physically vivacious the first 14 years I knew her and she has proved herself to be emotionally and mentally vivacious (as well as extraordinarily tough) for the past 13. Most of you would like her because she is a real person. She has survived – and many times thrived – because she is willing to struggle and scream and spit and cuss when her illness has brought her to the end of her tether. There's nothing phony about Sherrie or about her condition. Our story may not be pretty, but it is real.

The Four Phases

— *or* —

Journey to a Higher Level

Psychologists and management consultants have long studied group dynamics. They have found that when groups of people evolve to higher levels of communication and effectiveness, they tend to do so in four fairly predictable phases. Noted author and psychologist M. Scott Peck wrote about these phases in a book titled, *A World Waiting to be Born: Civility Rediscovered.*

I often refer to those four phases in my work with corporate executives and employees. I have also found that families and individuals tend to relate to each other primarily in one of the four phases. As I started to write this book, I realized that my evolution in handling Sherrie's illness also was tied directly to these phases. Therefore, I use them as a framework upon which the book is structured. Section one includes essays that explain how I handled Sherrie's illness and my relationship with her while operating primarily in phase one – known as the pseudo-community phase. Section two relates to phase two or the chaos phase, and so on.

Peck and others find that most organizations and work teams only bounce back and forth between the first two phases of pseudo-community and chaos. My work with corporate groups confirms that finding. An invisible barrier prevents most groups of people, including families, from operating at the higher levels of phases three and four, which are referred to as the phases of emptiness and community, respectively. The barbs of this barrier include discomfort, something most of us choose to bypass if possible. When I describe the four phases to groups, I often write attributes of each phase on a flip chart, starting with the attributes of phase one at the bottom of the page, and working my way up to the attributes of phase four at the top of the page. I then draw a barbed wire across the center of the page, separating phases one and two from phases three and four. I will occasionally refer to operating "above or below the barbed wire" Regrettably, most groups and individuals operate below the barrier.

One benefit of Sherrie's ongoing illness is that it has helped to force me to break through that barbed wire, to go above it. Chronic illness continues to put hurdles in our lives, but it also brought Sherrie and me closer than I imagined possible. By reading the following essays you will see how we made the progression from phase one's pseudo-community to the community of phase four. Below is a brief description of each phase.

Phase One – Pseudo-community (Plastic People)
People who display behavior patterns characteristic of phase one wear masks, usually of the happy-face variety. They avoid conflict, often at all costs. They pretend life is not difficult and they seek to avoid discomfort, even if it means facing bigger problems in the future. Phase one is a charade. People who operate in this phase think that by being nice and polite they become an effective team. That's bull! Groups (or families or

couples) that operate in the pseudo-community phase are far less effective than they could be. They refrain from showing any true emotion, which is one reason this phase reeks of dishonesty. Niceness, comfort and dishonesty are characteristic attributes of people who dwell in phase one.

Phase Two – Chaos (Angry People)

Phase one people hold in their emotions. The group moves to phase two from phase one usually when emotional outbursts occur. Their masks crack in this phase and emotions sometimes come streaming forth. However, chaos can emerge in less dramatic ways, too, such as by forming coalitions or using passive-aggressive language, which I call "coward talk." Conflict often sparks a group to move to this phase. Unfortunately, group members approach problems with a win-lose mentality instead of seeking the best group decision. Conflict becomes personal. Chaos is also a formula for dishonesty and ineffectiveness. However, Peck and others believe groups must go through phase two if they hope to reach phase four. While chaos sounds ugly, groups can move into this important phase in a way that does not cut others to shreds. Section two of this book describes how that can happen. Anger, back biting and win-lose thinking are characteristic attributes of people who dwell in phase two.

Phase Three – Emptiness (Vulnerable People)

The masks come off in this phase. People get fed up with the charade and anger of the first two phases. One or more people start telling the truth from both the mind and heart. They display the courage to become vulnerable. Catastrophe can also move a group (or family) into this phase. Silence is common in phase three, and during that silence, insight and connection often bloom. Emptiness evokes emotions such as empathy, a definite human trait. In emptiness, people revel in their humanness rather than denying it as in phase one. Once the masks and fear of vulnerability leave, group or family members become truly honest. There is recognition that life is difficult. People in emptiness are willing to move ahead, no matter what the circumstances. Vulnerability, honesty and human connections are characteristic attributes of people who dwell in phase three.

Phase Four – Community (Real People)

People who have reached phase four have started to build true relationships. They view others as real people rather than as job titles or labels. The thought of wearing masks is horrible and even laughable to people who have entered the community phase. They know life is difficult and address problems head-on, with honesty. Community members seek win-win solutions. They believe feelings are neither right nor wrong, they just are. Therefore, they illuminate conversation by sharing their emotions honestly. Unlike the first two phases, people in phase four are honest and primed to be more effective. They also have greater satisfaction because they do not have to play charades or take everything so personally. Honesty, conflict resolution and relationships are characteristic attributes of those who reach phase four.

There's a good chance that you and a loved one approach chronic illness while you are still residing in phases one and two. This makes a bad situation even worse. Read the following essays to see how to journey through the illness and live at a higher level.

The Primary Cast of Characters

— or —

My Family

This book focuses primarily on my approach to Sherrie's chronic illness. While I refer to parents, friends, co-workers and doctors, among others, my nuclear family colors all aspects of this book and my life. Therefore, here's a brief glance at the five members of my family.

Sherrie

Born June 15, 1953, in Longmont, Colo., Sherrie grew up an athletic tomboy and, unfortunately, finished high school two years before the state of Colorado sponsored girls' sports. Nevertheless, her love of sports led her to acquire a physical education degree – with an adult-fitness concentration – from Colorado State University (CSU) in 1978. Sherrie enjoys singing and acting when her health permits. She is a full-time homemaker and is a trusted confidante of both our kids and their friends. Sherrie and I married on Aug. 19, 1973.

Corlet (pronounced Core-lay)

Born Dec. 30, 1980, in Loveland, Colo., our daughter Corlet will graduate from high school in 1999 and attend college or a fashion-design school. Her main loves are her friends, her boyfriend – Matt – and a funky 1984 Volvo station wagon plastered with strange stickers.

Alyse

Born Nov. 8, 1982, in Loveland, Colo., our daughter Alyse plans to graduate from high school in 2001 and attend college. She participates in cross-country running and basketball at school. When not playing sports, she loves to hang out with friends.

Bret

Born Oct. 5, 1988, in Colorado Springs, Colo., Bret was adopted by Sherrie and me when he was three days old. Bret also loves sports of all kinds and hopes to one day be a professional soccer player, artist or forest ranger.

Gregg

Born Nov. 21, 1950, in Omaha, Neb., I'm a former jock who married my semi-pro baseball teammate's sister. I grew up in Boulder, Colo., and earned a journalism degree from CSU in 1975. I'm a former award-winning journalist and public relations manager who now owns Leader's Edge Consulting, Inc. I use facilitation, training and coaching skills to help corporate managers and teams be more effective and satisfied. I also write a monthly leadership column for a regional business magazine.

References to others

I use only first names to describe friends and acquaintances in this book. In certain cases, I use false names to maintain the anonymity of certain people and let the reader know when I do so.

A Note From Sherrie

— *or* —

Exposing "The Lie"

Seeing this book come to fruition makes me glad that I did not listen to the lie in my head that told me my family would be better off without me. I hope that by reading how my husband and I dealt with my condition, couples and families will be inspired to do the hard work necessary to stay together and fight the battle against chronic illness as they grow in emotional, mental and spiritual strength.

I believe Gregg's book also offers those of us who are ill an opportunity to look outside ourselves and into the angst of those who love us most – our families and friends. One key message I read in *Beyond Chaos* is to allow ourselves to give and receive the love of friends and family – not by performing or competing for it, but by embracing each other in our weaknesses. If nothing else, I pray that readers will realize they are not alone in their struggles; there is hope.

— *Sherrie Piburn*

Acknowledgments

— *or* —

Kicking Into a Higher Gear

As my wife came to the final turn, the Death Valley of the 440-yard dash, two women with slim bodies nipped at her heels. The other women's slender legs stretched, hit and glided in unison. Sherrie's legs were more muscular in shape, causing little explosions of cinder dust as they pounded down the track.

All three women were dead-even into the 40-yard straight-away, until Sherrie kicked into a gear I didn't know she had. She broke the tape five yards ahead of her opponents. The next day the local newspaper ran a photo of my 25-year-old wife crossing the finish line with the anguished expression of a woman in childbirth. Sherrie won a tacky Loveland Superstars blue ribbon.

I can't tell you the exact day the wife of my youth died because her death didn't come nicely packaged with an obituary, a coffin or a hefty check from the insurance guy. Sherrie still lives, but the woman I married, the Sherrie who won races and climbed mountains, doesn't. Once I mentally put "the healthy Sherrie" to rest and grieved that loss, then and only then, was I able to journey with Sherrie beyond the Death Valley of our marriage and our lives.

I have three great children, wonderful parents, a support-ive brother and sister-in-law, a tough mother-in-law and sev-eral crazy and courageous buddies. I especially thank my buddy John for his honesty and support through the years. But when it comes to acknowledging those who have seen me through the writing of this book, I have to focus on Sherrie. Although this work is not primarily about Sherrie and her illness, but about me and the way I handled her maladies, anything writ-ten about me is both directly and indirectly about Sherrie as well. Thank you Sherrie, for your love and encouragement to write this book.

I also thank the Arthritis Foundation for having the courage to publish a work that strays from the typical self-help mold. Special thanks go to Beth Axtell and Sara Horton who offered insightful guidance and emotional support, which are equally appreciated.

A HAPPY-FACE MINDSET

(phase one **Pseudo-community.** Populated
by plastic people. Epitomized by
niceness, comfort, dishonesty.)

"*There, there, everything's
going to be OK.*"

chapter 1

LIFE'S A BREEZE

This chapter sets the historical context for
the rest of the book.

The Blank Canvas

— *or* —

Kindergarten Hell

When it comes to pure scared-out-of-my-wits-I-think-I'm-a-goner fear, my first day of kindergarten comes to mind. If life is a master artist, young children serve as its blank canvas. With each new experience, each new brush stroke, the artist – life – creates a child's mental image of his surroundings. Each canvas, of course, is unique.

The summer of 1956, I heard strange rumors that I would soon be heading off to a wonderful place called kindergarten. My life canvas up to that point conveyed messages of comfort and conformity. I tensed up thinking about changing my untroubled routine. Dad worked long and hard throughout the year. Brother Mike spent summers on our grandparents' farm and went to school when the new school term began. That left Mom and me together 24 hours a day, seven days a week.

A few days before I started kindergarten, Mom bought me new shoes, pants and a jacket. They were exciting reminders that a mysterious new chapter in my life was about to begin. But one overriding thought kept me from developing a preschool ulcer: Mom would be alongside me in this unknown land. She would protect me from danger and discomfort. I rarely left her sight – which is how both of us wanted it – and I had no clue that would change.

The big day arrived and Dad took the obligatory snapshot of me standing on the front sidewalk, ready to walk the three blocks to Bertha Barber Elementary School in Bellevue, Neb. Minutes later, Mom and I began our trek to school and I felt my heart racing. The "Great Unknown" felt terrifying and exciting at the same time. "Whoa," I thought, "Mom and I will be in kindergarten this year." When we entered the kindergarten classroom 10 minutes later, the sights and sounds of 22 kids jammed into a colorful room of bulletin boards and sparkling desks hit me like a Picasso abstract. I froze in my tracks, mystified by this fantastic part of life previously hidden from me.

After a few minutes my head cleared enough to logically make out what was happening. What I saw was a frenzy of kids, a calm, slender woman I correctly guessed was the teacher, and two or three other moms. Hey, wait a minute, where were the other moms? Hey, wait a gosh-darn minute, where was my Mom!? I turned to see her tiptoeing toward the exit. My leaden feet grew wings.

Showing the potential of a future Cornhusker linebacker, I grabbed onto Mom's coat and then began to screech and holler. No way was I doing this kindergarten thing alone. The teacher and Mom both tried to pry my fingers off Mom's coat. They shooshed me a million times, but I continued to bellow "No! No! No!" That minute of shooshes and shouts seemed to last a decade. The raucous standoff abruptly ended when I threw up on the floor. My classmates stood dumbfounded.

I might have lost my head of steam after vomiting, but not my conviction to go home. I settled down long enough for

Mom to call Dad, who worked 30 minutes away. He came, and in his manly way coaxed me into getting my act together. The script for my life had changed so much in that horrendous morning that there was no real chance of that ever happening. Dad drove Mom and me home before morning recess. I would have to venture to kindergarten another day.

Television helps paint the canvas of the mind of many youngsters. Most baby boomers learned that the Nelson family in the hit TV show had their act together. Comfort, consistency and an amazing lack of tough issues added up to smooth sailing for Ozzie, Harriet, David and Ricky. About 25 years later, another sit-com family pushed its way into American living rooms. The "Roseanne" show revealed the fictional Connor family traveling a rocky road compared to the smooth-sailing of the Nelsons. Discomfort, chaos and tough issues ruled Roseanne's roost. The common mindset of many viewers was that the Nelsons were healthy, the Connors, unhealthy. That perception represented my assessment of the two families, too, until I learned the hard lessons of chronic illness. My new assessment is that the Nelsons were in the dark, while the Connors were in the light. The Nelsons were unreal, the Connors, real.

My childhood canvas showed endless days of comfort interrupted by rare blips of difficulties. I learned early on that problems were abnormal and short-lived. Hey, I had a great childhood but, unfortunately, entered the adult years ill-prepared for life's challenges. The abstract Picasso brush strokes of a problem-filled life seemed obnoxiously foreign to the serene canvas of my comfortable life. Kindergarten and Sherrie's chronic illness blind-sided me. I didn't know how to deal with either. I didn't know how to talk about them. I never thought Sherrie would be sick for long. I always thought our problems would be short-lived. I assumed somebody – doctors, researchers, Lady Luck – would save the day. Unfortunately . . . and fortunately, they could not.

Life is Easy

— *or* —

Life is Difficult

L ike many people, I grew up with an invisible handicap. Thousands of people have read M. Scott Peck's best seller *The Road Less Traveled*. It remains popular 20 years after its first printing. Peck's opening line is as unforgettable and powerful as a swift jab to the nose. "Life is difficult" is what the first line of the book says. If boxing is the "sweet science," then Peck's three words represent sweet writing and powerful psychology. It's tough, effective, straight to the point.

Life is difficult. Before summer vacation started, Coach Foster told me to pump weights and put on 10 pounds. He expected me to be his starting tight end for the Fairview Knights my junior year of high school. I played baseball that summer, but failed to lift a single dumbbell or add a single pound. I assumed my natural ability would be sufficient. The night before those awful pre-season football practices started, I recalled the sweat and exhaustion of the previous year. Sitting in my parents' stuffy living room, I remembered the practice sessions when I dragged myself to bed at 7:00 every night. The thought of going through that difficulty again seemed abhorrent to me. I called Coach Foster at home and told him I wanted to focus on basketball and baseball and skip the football season that year. I didn't tell him the truth; football is too difficult.

That year, Fairview went to the state championship game while I sat in the press box, keeping statistics and hating myself.

"Once we truly know that life is difficult – once we truly understand and accept it – then life is no longer difficult," Peck writes. "Because once it is accepted, the fact that life is difficult no longer matters."

I spent 30 years or so of my life assuming life was meant to be easy. In general, it had been. I assumed it would continue to be so. Oh, I occasionally heard gray-haired types saying everyone would have to pay their dues eventually, but I assumed I would be able to go through the game of life without having to pay for the ticket. Of course, there's another message embedded in this paragraph. Spectators worry about tickets. Participants play the damn game. Sixty or so of my peers on my high school's 1967-68 football team chose the difficult road and participated in a glorious Cinderella season. I chose comfort, and watched a storybook season from the sanitary confines of the press box.

A 76-year study conducted by the University of California, Riverside, presents a surprising theory on human longevity. Over the course of the study, some participants died relatively young, while others still live. It was found that among the group studied, people who grew up in idyllic childhood settings, where life was "easy," tended to die early. Those who had a difficult childhood generally lived longer. Apparently, the latter group learned early on that life was difficult and developed ways to handle or resolve tough issues.

Peck writes: "Life is a series of problems. Do we want to moan about them or solve them?" I get the feeling those who lived to become old-timers in the study mentioned above chose to solve their problems. As a person who thought life should be easy, I more often moaned about them. I thought life was supposed to be easy because my childhood was so easy.

In 1980 I was forced to face the difficulty of life. Corlet's birth was imminent. Sherrie and I were about to become parents. And I was about to become unemployed. I had worked for a company that produced motivational and educational audio tapes. But after six months I realized no more paychecks would be coming. I said good-bye to my boss and prepared for job hunting and parenting. Corlet came into our lives a week later. For two months I searched for a job while also getting to know my little daughter. When I received a job offer from a reputable Fortune 100 company, I nearly collapsed in relief. I told myself I would never have to look for a job again. "They'll either give me a gold watch when I'm 70 or carry me out of the plant in a coffin," I thought. I wanted job security, I wanted career comfort, I wanted ease over difficulty, I wanted stagnation over growth.

So why do I tell you all of this? Because it sets the context for the rest of the book. Like many people, I believed life should be easy. A lifetime of choosing comfort over discomfort at all costs prevented me from being able to confront problems effectively when they came. But the biggest difficulty, the issue that changed my family's life more than any other, did not occur until my mid-30s. That was when my gorgeous and vibrant wife of 11 years became chronically ill.

This book is about my journey of grief and growth while responding to her illness. It's about getting "beyond chaos" in coping with my wife's chronic illness. It's about me learning to cope with a difficult life. Ben Franklin said, "Those things that hurt, instruct." This book is not about making victims of those of us who live with people who are chronically ill. America's roll call of victim groups spills over the brim already. This is a book about how to stand up to chronic illness, "The Intruder," which presents opportunities to both grieve and to grow.

Jocks Made in Heaven

— or —

Losing the "Sweet Spot"

Sherrie, a slender, blonde girl with large hazel eyes appeared more fragile than ferocious. Neighbors often saw laughing boys chasing her from yard to yard. Occasionally, she would downshift, letting a boy catch her. If it was the boy's first time to tackle her, he soon learned a shocking fact: Sherrie had the soul of a gruff-voiced professional wrestler. She would escape the boy's grasp with her fists flying, then pin his shoulders to the ground.

The shy, skinny boy who had panicked in kindergarten discovered a startling fact on the playground: I could run faster, jump higher and throw farther than any of my classmates. Although classroom learning came easily to me, so much so that I became one of the top students in elementary school, the playground became my realm. It was the place where that best part of me could burst forth and be known to others and myself.

Close your eyes and envision a blank canvas. Then begin to paint a picture of who or what you are. What emerges? The best pianist at school? A business manager? The fastest runner in the county? An artist? A dad? A mom? Without consciously thinking about it often, humans constantly seek to define themselves. Kids have a special need to begin to paint a mental picture of who and what they are.

Young Sherrie's painting would have shown a tough, fast body zig-zagging through angry streaks of multicolored brush strokes. The scene is chaotic, but the message is clear: That lithe body has the potential to break free from her stormy childhood home. My childhood painting would have been far less eye-catching than Sherrie's image. Straight lines interspersed with dull colors. That part of the painting symbolizes my shyness and the predictability of my life. But one corner of the canvas would have shown a sinewy athlete racing toward a sunrise. That one corner gave life – and hope – to the painting.

As a teenager, Sherrie's legs grew thick and muscular while increasing their feminine appeal. She used those legs to literally escape from the discord of home and school life in Longmont, Colo. An avid Girl Scout, Sherrie spent many weekends on long treks through the nearby Rocky Mountains. Her physical life provided her with a positive self-image and a means of escape.

Boulder, Colo., in the 1960s presented a perfect playground for sexual and political revolutionaries. I failed to fit the mold of that decadent decade. I did not outshine all others in sports, but I still excelled and my spirit soared on athletic fields.

Sherrie and I grew up within a half-marathon of each other. Her home life was a frantic two-minute drill on the gridiron, mine, a long doubleheader in mid-August. We each looked to our respective bodies for self-image and hope.

I saw a beautiful, tanned girl approach the fence near the on-deck circle. The young woman whispered something to my teammate, Jerry. An inning later I asked Jerry who the girl was. "My sister, Sherrie," said Jerry, the shortstop on this semi-pro baseball team. A week later, after a July 4, 1971, doubleheader, Jerry and I went on a double date with Sherrie and another woman.

Two weeks later Sherrie and I went on our first solo date. We spent a summer evening walking up and down the streets of Estes Park, a mountain resort community. On the way home, we stopped for a short hike in the woods and a first kiss. I ended up marrying the shortstop's sister. "Baze-uh-ball haz bin berry berry gewd to me."

Every baseball player knows about "the sweet spot," which is that part of the bat that packs the most power. A list of famous "sweet spots" includes Albert Einstein's brain, Mother Teresa's heart, Jerry Seinfeld's humor, Barbra Streisand's voice and John Elway's arm. Sherrie's and my "sweet spots" were our physically fit bodies. We each depended on our own bodies and liked what we saw of the other's.

Imagine Einstein with Alzheimer's disease. Picture a selfish Mother Teresa or a dead-serious Jerry Seinfeld as an account rep in a purchasing department. Give Barbra Streisand permanent laryngitis. Try to transform John Elway into a defensive lineman. The pictures ain't pretty. Sherrie lost her "sweet spot" when chronic illness came to town. Gregg's "sweet spot" became weaker indirectly as a result of Sherrie's illness.

Some people lose their "sweet spots" and slowly deteriorate. Others look for and develop new ones so the image on their canvas of life changes. Many relationships (including marriages and friendships) disintegrate during struggles with chronic illness. Perhaps people cling too long to the old images. Sherrie and I clung to the old images and struggled mightily. Eventually and thankfully, the images changed. For both of us, a few rays of light began to appear on the canvases.

Richard Nixon & Barney Fife

— *or* —

The Honeymoon & "The Intruder"

I stood in front of JC Penney at a shopping center in Boulder, Colo. I expected my green 1964 Chevy Impala to appear any time. I had lent the car to Sherrie, my fiancée of five weeks. Our wedding was two days away. After five minutes, I saw what looked to be my car coming slowly toward me. As it drew closer, however, I saw an unrecognizable head of hair. Sherrie had long auburn hair. The driver heading my way had short-cropped hair. It looked like a young man behind the wheel. Still, it looked like my car.

The Impala stopped at the curb and I slowly walked toward it, bending down slightly to get a look at who I presumed to be a thief behind the wheel. I wondered if the driver had thrown my beautiful fiancée into the trunk. I peered into the window and saw the wrong hair but the right face. "Get in," Sherrie said matter-of-factly, forgetting she looked like her mythical twin brother.

Without saying a word, Sherrie's haircut conveyed the message that she might become my wife, but she would definitely continue to do things her way. She need not ask permission. In the springtime of our lives, that message of personal freedom rang true for me, too. Shoot, I fell in love with Sherrie partially because of her willingness to buck trends and follow her heart.

Fast-forward to the future: Heavy footsteps thud down the hallway from our bedroom. Sherrie staggers into the kitchen, looking the part of a suburban lush. "Cyall shuh poishun shenter!" I ask, "Huh?"

As a twosome, we bucked several traditional wedding trends to the dismay of our parents. Instead of a white gown, Sherrie wore a low-cut black dress. Instead of a tuxedo, I wore a paisley shirt and leather vest. Hey, it was the Age of Aquarius! Instead of having Aunt Martha play the organ, we hired a stranger to play a flute-like recorder. We gave the pastor permission to wear a Nehru jacket.

We got hitched without a hitch, despite looking like the cast from "Laugh-In." We had one more wedding tradition to break. Instead of flying to Mexico or staying in a nice hotel closer to home, we chose to backpack across the Continental Divide to celebrate our honeymoon. No boundaries, no money, no champagne, no solid food, no bed. We had each other and the packs on our back. We also had an erroneous view of what life might throw our way. In that season of our lives, when we thought we knew everything there was to know about anything, we thought life was at our disposal.

Fast-forward to the future: Sherrie lunges for a piece of paper beside the phone and smacks a finger on the printing. "Shuh poishun shenter!" I fumble the phone. I was jittery Deputy Barney Fife grasping for his one damn bullet.

I snapped a picture of my gorgeous, short-haired wife on the first day of our marriage, the first day of our honeymoon trek. The photo shows Sherrie squirting water from a goat-skin flask into her mouth. Her profile reveals muscular arms and legs capable of hiking 20 miles per day on rocky terrain 12,000 feet above sea level. Moments after clicking the shutter, before we headed farther up the trail, we said something I'll always regret. It was akin to Nixon saying, "I'm not a crook!"

"You know," I said in an exaggeratedly deep voice, "when you've got your health, you've got just about everything." Sherrie chuckled and said, "Yep, everything." Those words, as did Nixon's, came back to haunt us. On that August day in 1973, you could have told us a U.S. president would resign within the decade and we could have hesitantly accepted that prediction. You might have said that the USSR would crumble before the turn of the century, and we could have bought it. You could have told us we would one day own a small oven that cooks food in seconds, and we would have nodded our approval. But if you had told us that day, atop the Divide, that one of us would become chronically ill in his or her 30s, we would have laughed in your face. You would have gotten the same reaction from us if you had predicted aliens would land on the White House lawn in 1998. After laughing, we would have hoisted our heavy packs onto our backs and marched up the mountain, away from you and your silly little comment.

Fast-forward to the future: I finally reach a poison expert by phone and hear that I should induce vomiting in case a concoction of prescribed drugs has backfired. We later find out a strain of Asian flu is the cause of Sherrie's slurred speech that night. Flu or not, Sherrie's symptoms of pain, headaches, exhaustion and depression continue.

Chronic illness acts as a thief in the night. We thought our great health and exercise regimen served as an impenetrable security system to thwart that intruder. In our minds, the odds of getting zapped by a lightning bolt were greater than one of us getting sick for more than a week. When "The Intruder" entered the open window of our lives we were dumbstruck. We refused to believe the reality of the theft. "The Intruder" took many things, including Sherrie's good health and a fair chunk of our freedom and fun. We kept waiting for the earth to get back on its regular orbit around the sun so things would go back to being normal, healthy, fun. It took a long time for us to fully comprehend that "The Intruder" had slipped into our lives, robbed us and eluded the cops.

The whole experience taught us many things. It also taught us one thing. "When you've got your health, you've got just about everything."

Ambushed North of the Border

— or —

Embarking on a Different Journey

The year was 1985. I felt entrenched in my job, as if stuck in a thick bowl of gravy. That made sense, since it was the quintessential "gravy" job. As public relations manager for a large division of a Fortune 100 company, I had some community clout without many concrete commitments to fulfill. However, four years into this mundane position, I desperately needed a diversion. Sherrie needed one, too. Sherrie had quit her job as a full-time wellness director before Corlet was born in 1980. Two years later, Alyse came along. Sherrie didn't bounce back from this delivery, feeling for months as if her energy level ran near empty. Despite the malaise, she continued to work part time, teaching several aerobics and cardiac rehabilitation classes weekly. She also taught cross-country skiing some weekends.

Twelve years of marriage had dulled some of our honeymoon dreams. In 1985, Sherrie and I realized we had allowed society to put boundaries on us. We were living the standard-fare, mid-'80s, baby-boomer-gone-stale life of the suburbs. In '72 I voted McGovern. In '84 I cast my ballot for Reagan. Enough said. We needed a personal revolution but chose the safer route. We decided that our safer route translated itself into our taking a summer sabbatical in Mexico. Sherrie longed to return to Mexico City where she had spent two weeks during a Girl

Scout trip in high school. I did not share that longing, but decided to check out possibilities to get us there.

First, I received permission from my boss to take a three-month leave of absence – without pay. Then I began searching for opportunities to put my journalistic skills to work south of the border. Our church has missionaries working throughout the world, including Mexico City. I contacted the denomination headquarters in Chicago, and after discussing my trip with the church leaders they expressed an interest in having me write magazine articles and develop a slide show about the people and activities of that particular mission.

A week later, the denomination's officials agreed on my responsibilities and the stipend I would receive in exchange for my work. The church located a trailer where my family and I would live. The officials also said we would have to drive, rather than fly to Mexico City because I would need a car to carry out my duties. As the details of the trip became more clear, Sherrie felt energized; I, on the other hand, grew more tense. (I'll tell you more about that in a later chapter.) Our girls knew little of the trip's specifics, but sensed they were going on an adventure.

A week before we embarked on that adventure designed for people free of real or unreal limits, Sherrie came down with flu-like symptoms marked by terrible nausea. The last thing you want to do while battling nausea is begin a days-long drive through the desert of the Southwest and Mexico. So, I called our church headquarters in Chicago to say we would postpone our departure by a week. To put it bluntly, the following week Sherrie still felt like crap. She was still experiencing nausea, now coupled with migraine and exhaustion. We postponed the trip for another week.

About a month later, we canceled the trip altogether and I went back to work. We saw no improvement in Sherrie's condition and realized our summer break would not occur in 1985. In truth, Sherrie's ongoing illness not only prevented us from going that year, but also kept us from even thinking about such a journey. Mexico City vanished from our vocabulary and our plans, only to be replaced by the words doctors and specialists as we started a long and arduous venture along the uncharted path of chronic illness where we sought answers rather than adventure.

I speak only a bit of Spanish. However, I would have had more luck asking street directions from a native of Mexico City than getting answers from the first set of medical professionals we approached. Sherrie's illness baffled our doctors. They scratched their heads and shrugged their shoulders. They sometimes gave pat answers based on their specialty or mumbled something about the two of us needing to try marriage counseling to get Sherrie out of her malaise.

Hey, it should not be this hard to find answers, I thought. Amazingly, no doctors or researchers stepped forward with a decent diagnosis, let alone a prognosis. Lady Luck was a no-show, too, but another fine lady, who is real, showed us a possible course of action. My Great Aunt Wilma, who lives in Shenandoah, Iowa, sent us an *Omaha World-Herald* newspaper article about chronic fatigue syndrome (CFS). It described symptoms similar to Sherrie's. At long last we had a possible name to apply to this mysterious enemy. In addition, the article quoted a doctor said to be one of the world's CFS experts. Our luck was changing – the doctor practiced medicine in Denver, an hour from our home.

BEYOND CHAOS

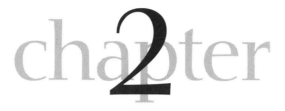

chapter 2

THE "BIG 5" IN
PHASE ONE

I selected five major topics to discuss in the
second chapter of each section. The topics
are: support, the medical maze, parenting,
intimacy and spirituality. By reading the whole
book you will see how I progressed through
the four phases in dealing with these topics.

Support:
Sticky Labels, Mental Chains

— or —

Be Set Free

I stood in front of 25 corporate employees who came to hear my presentation titled, "Coping with Chronic Illness and the Labels it Creates." Approximately half the group had some form of chronic illness while the other half supported a loved one who was ill. Being in a corporate setting, I asked the group to name the duties and personality profile of a typical general manager within that company. This served as a mental warm-up for the next activity. After a minute of mental "calisthenics," I went to the flip chart and wrote the word "patient" on a sheet of paper. On another flip chart nearby, I wrote the word "caretaker." I explained that the word "patient" referred to people who are chronically ill, while the word "caretaker" was a label for those people who love and support "patients." I said, "Let's brainstorm society's view of the roles and personalities of these two 'jobs.'" I wrote their responses on the flip chart pages.

"PATIENT"	"CARETAKER"
Depressed	Burdened
Restricted	A saint
Whiny	Supportive
Unpredictable	Overprotective
Frustrated	Co-dependent
Exhausted	Confused
Inadequate	Tireless
Dependent	Selfless
Searching	A martyr
	Uncomplaining
	Stoical

The words came fast and furiously. They knew what society expected of these two "jobs." My theory is that audience members whipped the words out quickly because they also lived them. America seems enthralled by labels. They represent an easy short-cut for describing and categorizing people. Think of the following labels we put on people.

**Celebrity • Drunkard • Jock
Intellectual • Stud • Nerd**

When I read these words, pictures come to mind of what people under each label look and sound like. I have a clear mental picture of how they live, based on stereotypes and generalizations bandied about in society. Of course the generalizations and stereotypes used by people are often incorrect. Not all drunkards have two-day stubble and live on the streets. Not all intellectuals are liberal college professors who have emaciated bodies and the social acumen of a badger. One reason I left the corporate world to start a one-man consulting business is that I hate to box myself into a job title. I love my freedom. Labels, in subtle and not-so-subtle ways, hinder one's freedom to be oneself.

Go back to the "job descriptions" for "patients" and "caretakers." I find both lists repulsive. How would you like to think of yourself as whiny, depressed and dependent or as a burdened saint or a tireless martyr? The more others expect you to live by those labels, the more likely you are to begin thinking that is your proper role. Even worse, you become that label personified. Similarly, think how dangerous it is to expect a loved one to live by those inane descriptors. If you spend months and months thinking of your significant other as whiny, depressed and dependent or as a burdened saint and a tireless martyr, it might become reality in both of your minds.

I confess that I put a label of "patient" on Sherrie and "caretaker" on myself. Those labels prevented me from moving forward truthfully, creatively and lovingly. Sherrie became wrapped in a sticky label with words such as "fragile" and "moody" and "China doll." She was no longer just Sherrie. The label overpowered in my mind the true essence of who she was. I saw her differently and started to treat her differently. Naturally, my words and actions matched the "caretaker's" roles and personality. I became the stoical martyr whose job was to keep all the plates spinning on the little sticks.

Study the words listed under the labels above. By living up to them, my relationship with Sherrie, and hers with me, became utilitarian rather than joyful. We did our duties rather than responding to each other in true love. Look how nicely the dysfunctional characteristics of each "job" fit together like pieces of a puzzle. In some partnerships, they fit so nicely that it seems perfectly natural to continue living by the labels for years.

Exhausted — Tireless
Restricted — Overprotective
Dependent — Co-dependent

Over time, Sherrie and I found that we had boxed ourselves in individually to our "job" descriptions – literally and figuratively. And when we finally realized what we had done to ourselves, we destroyed the labels and felt as if we had just busted out of solitary confinement. We are no longer two individuals marching to the duties of our labels, but two people who simply love each other. It opened up new avenues for how we responded to the good and bad days.

The more I thought about labels – even outside of the context of chronic illness – the more I chose to obliterate them. A buddy helped me realize how to do that. A college English professor, Andy is the smartest person I know. One day while we walked through a sunlit park, he said: "I could consider myself an intellectual, but I prefer to tell myself and others that I enjoy intellectual pursuits." It made perfect sense. To wrap Andy inside the intellectual label would be to belittle the many other true and strong aspects of his life. Here is a crazy guy who looks like a movie star, loves his family, plays by his own set of rules, is a physical rock and enjoys intellectual pursuits.

Many of the following essays tell stories about how I screwed up when I tried to be a stoical martyr or saint in dealing with Sherrie's chronic illness. In the essays, you will also see how things went much better for Sherrie and me when I trashed the "caretaker" and "patient" label. Trashing the labels didn't mean that I planned to ignore my appropriate responsibilities. What it means however, is that I want to enjoy life and address challenges outside the confines of sticky labels. I ripped them from my psyche, and I suggest you do the same. Be set free.

note I refrain from using labels such as "caretaker" and "patient" in this book. When they appear, I put quotation marks around them to remind readers that I do not like them or the stereotypes they support. Instead, I typically use phrases such as "a person who is chronically ill and the people who love them." In addition, I do not refer to professional caretakers when I use the term "caretaker."

Medical Maze:
Join the Medical Team

— *or* —

Be Weird and Compassionate

Raise your hand if you enjoy waiting in a doctor's reception area. Raise your other hand if you enjoy waiting some more once situated in a doctor's exam room. Now, for those one or two people in the universe who have both hands raised, you are in the surrender posture. A cop should now cuff you and haul you off to Weird Jail.

Look, the only reason most of us put up with a long wait in the doctor's office is because we have a health problem that needs to be addressed. Some people look for ridiculous excuses to bypass going to the doctor's office even when they know their problem will not go away on its own. So, if some humans refrain from making doctor appointments for themselves, why would anyone go to someone else's appointment? Only weird people would volunteer for such unpleasant duty, right? Well, weird or compassionate people.

In the first 12 years of marriage, with the exception of family-oriented visits to the doctor, for example during Sherrie's pregnancies, Sherrie went to most of her doctors' appointments alone and I went to most of mine alone. On those occasions when we made a joint trip, we were looking forward to something POSITIVE, such as cute little babies, rather than dwelling on something NEGATIVE, like a mysterious, long-term illness. In those first six months of Sherrie's illness, when we were searching for a diagnosis, I went to some of her appointments. But not all. Hey, I had a full-time job and we were a single-income family.

OK, OK. I rarely did anything truly important or meaningful at my corporate job and I never lost income by going with Sherrie. It sounded like a great excuse but, at least in my case, it didn't hold water. In reality, I just didn't want to go. I also questioned my value in going. I didn't know the right words to say to Sherrie before or after the appointment, and most of the time when I accompanied her, I sat like a bump on a log. In the early days of Sherrie's illness I subscribed to the philosophy that we listened, doctors talked. We had unspoken questions, they had spoken and unspoken answers. We were needy, they were saviors. We were dumb, they were brilliant. I generally try to stay away from places in which I feel needy and dumb.

Therefore, Sherrie would head into this onerous and confusing maze of doctors' offices on her own, while I did truly important stuff at the office such as read junk mail, call my buddy at a nearby division, and eat lunch at the cafeteria. That night, if I remembered Sherrie had gone to visit a doctor, I would ask how it went. In the initial period of her illness, Sherrie's condition included cloudy thinking. Her brain just wasn't its normal sharp self. She had a hard time telling me what the doctor said. I would get huffy and my non-verbal retort was: "Well, gee, why are we spending all this money on doctors if you can't even remember what they said?" You're right, I was a jerk.

As I've progressed in this journey, I've changed my philosophy. If possible, I now go with Sherrie to her appointments. Not only can I help clarify the communication between Sherrie and the doctor, I can also provide some moral support before, during and after the appointment. For those of you willing to be weird or compassionate, here are five tips on how to make the appointments more valuable.

1. Help your significant other develop a list of questions to ask the doctor.

By putting your heads together you will likely develop a more comprehensive set of questions that will be important to ask the doctor. Make sure to take a written list of the questions to the appointment and be sure the doctor answers all of them. That frees up the ill person to respond to the doctor's questions and requests during the appointment.

2. Make sure your significant other writes down or knows the medications currently being used.

Doctors always ask Sherrie about her medications. Fortunately, she always knows in great detail what she is taking. Your significant other might not be so clear on that so help him or her by creating a list.

3. Make the appointment part of a weekday mini-date.

Doctors' appointments are not much fun. So make it part of a package deal. Go out to eat before or after the appointment. If you have the freedom to do so, plan to attend a matinee right after the visit to the doctor's office. Such a "date" also represents a way to celebrate good news at an appointment.

4. Be a facilitator of information.

You can play less of a neutral role if you act as facilitator during an appointment. For example, maybe the "patient" would never question a doctor's advice. That doesn't mean you can't. It might take a bit of courage for you to say, "Doctor, I believe your advice to do some moderate workouts caused some problems last month." That is information the doctor needs to hear from someone. On the other hand, your significant other might downplay certain symptoms. As facilitator, you might say, "I just want to remind you that last Saturday you were in so much pain you needed me to come out into the garage and carry that light bag of groceries into the kitchen." Again, you can shed additional light on important issues. The more illumination (key information communicated), the more helpful the appointment will be for everyone.

5. Provide gentle reminders.

Before the appointment ends, have the doctor summarize what the patient should do in the coming days. Write down the steps. Then – in as loving and supportive a way as possible – encourage your significant other to follow those steps.

From an old pseudo-community standpoint, doctors' appointments are a drag. Approached in a new way, with your presence and help, doctors' appointments can shed more light on an illness than ever before. The tangible results include more perceptive and helpful directions from the doctor because of the increased information you provide. The intangible results include a closer relationship between yourself and the person who is ill.

Parenting:
Keeping Kids in the Dark

— *or* —

When the Bogeyman Is You

C an you imagine jumping out of your 6-year-old daughter's closet five minutes after she's settled down for the night? You are wearing a werewolf mask and your blood-curdling scream shakes her out of her near slumber. Your arms and legs flail like a scarecrow's as you come near her bed. Her little eyes seem to pop from her face and her piercing scream harmonizes with your deep-pitched yell to create a grotesque cacophony of fear. You would have to be stupid or a sicko (or both) to do such a thing.

Yet, one day, I created in a far more subtle scene the same level of fear in my 6-year-old daughter. Since I had not broken out of the pseudo-community phase, I blame that insidious villain for playing a leading role in this incident. Remember, in phase one we avoid conflict, we hide behind masks, we squelch open and honest communication. In the pseudo-community phase, we play specific roles. Adults, for example, talk about adult things, while keeping kids in the dark about the events of the grown-up world.

Sherrie had gone to the hospital in 1987 for her second surgery, a hysterectomy, within the last year. We asked my parents to come early in the day so they could watch our two young daughters while I went to be with Sherrie. As if I didn't have enough on my mind, I also felt extreme pressure about work. Bottom line: I had way too many things on my plate.

By late morning, the surgery was over and the surgeon told me things went well. He suggested I go home for lunch since Sherrie was zoned out in the recovery room for another hour or two. I went home, feeling exhausted in my own "caretaker" way. I walked through the front door and saw Corlet and her 4-year-old sister, Alyse, playing in the family room. Dad was setting the dining-room table and Mom was fixing sandwiches for lunch. I was handling that day as I would a busy shift at work. My brain was operating on overdrive and I had given my heart the day off. As I mentally checked off items on my to-do list, I gave little or no thought to the concerns and feelings of those around me.

"How did it go?" my Mom asked. I told my parents the doctor said the operation went well. Then Mom asked for more details. I walked through the dining room into the family room. I patted each daughter on the head. "Well, let's see. We got her checked in by 7 a.m. Sherrie and I chatted in her room for about 30 minutes." I walked to the other side of the room to look through a pile of mail on my desk. "I think they put her to sleep around 9:00 or so."

A moment later I walked back to the dining room to help Dad finish setting the table. "C'mon, girls, it's time to eat," I said. I was a robot moving my family and myself through my DayTimer schedule. "Item 987: Get family and self to eat lunch."

We ate lunch quietly. We all seemed exhausted. Then, as Mom got up to begin putting dishes in the sink, Corlet looked at me with sorrowful eyes. "Did they put Mommy to sleep like they did to Boone?" Her words jolted my spirit like a Mike Tyson punch to the gut.

"Oh Lord, no, Corlet," I said with my first tinge of empathy all day. "Why did you say that?"

"You said they put Mommy to sleep about 9:00 and that is how they killed our old dog," she said in a small, strained voice.

"I'm sorry, Corlet. They gave her a shot so she would sleep through the operation and it would not hurt her," I said, trying to take the fear from her mind. Within seconds she and her kid sister were playing dolls again in the corner of the family room.

I thought how it must feel to hear your father say "they" put your mother to sleep like some old Labrador Retriever. It seemed especially strange that the father and grandparents seemed so calm about what appeared to be a tragic event in the mind of a child. I forgot my worries at work. I mentally trashed my idiotic to-do list. I sent my brain home early and asked my heart to take charge. I grabbed a doll and played with my daughters. Then, after a few minutes, I set each daughter on my lap and squeezed them ever so gently.

Intimacy:
Muffling the Parentheses
— *or* —
Relationship Killers

Lovers often perform sex in the dark, in the nighttime, with the lights turned off. In my professional writing and speaking I often use the term, "turn on the lights." It is my way to encourage open and honest communication in corporate settings. If life is difficult, you increase the odds of solving problems by handling them in the light rather than in the dark.

For the first 12 years of marriage, Sherrie and I had a relatively healthy and active sex life. True, we didn't talk much about what did or did not feel good. Occasionally Sherrie would say she preferred to simply cuddle, but in my naive, immature way I would turn on the charm or put on a pout and eventually get what I wanted. Open and honest communication about sex felt uncomfortable and, frankly, unnecessary. If we just let nature take its course everything would work out just fine – at least by my standards.

The plastic people of the pseudo-community phase revel in the world of niceness, comfort and dishonesty. Why go below the surface in communication when everything seems fine on the outside? Blam! Sherrie's illness erupted in the summer of 1985. People in phase one do not like change. They seek comfortable and predictable lives. You really mess with their minds when you rock the boat. Chronic illness rocked our boat in many ways, including sexually.

In pseudo-community, people tend to ignore or avoid conflict. It's just too darned uncomfortable to talk about it. Sherrie's health problems definitely rocked the boat that had been our comfortable and satisfying sex life. But, being good citizens of the happy and phony community that is phase one, we rarely talked about the new challenges to our sex life. Let's take a peek at the Piburns in those early years of Sherrie's illness.

Setting: *Gregg and Sherrie's bedroom. The lights are dim and the married couple lie in bed, not quite touching. They speak in hushed tones so as not to awaken any of the kids in nearby bedrooms. Their unspoken thoughts appear in parentheses.*

Gregg: So how are you feeling tonight? (Let's get it on!)

Sherrie: As usual, crappy. (Hours and hours of sleep are all I want.)

Gregg: But you seemed a little better today, am I right? (Let's get it on!)

Sherrie: Oh, maybe a little. (I've improved from shitty to crappy ... yippee!)

Gregg: I've really missed you, if you know what I mean. (Let's get it on!)

Sherrie: No, I guess I don't know exactly what you mean. (If it's "let's get it on!" we're both in trouble.)

Gregg: Oh, you know, a bit of lovemaking. (I'm needy. Work with me on this one, OK?)

Sherrie: Gregg, I miss our lovemaking so much but I just don't think my body can handle it tonight. (What I miss most of all is you wrapping your warm arms around me through the night.)

Gregg: OK. (Crap-oh-la!)

Sherrie: Are you sure it's OK? (C'mon, Gregg, tell me what's really on your mind.)

Gregg: Yeah, I'm OK. I'm just sorry you feel so lousy every day and every night. (When will this nightmare ever end?)

Sherrie: I'm sorry, too. (I feel so damned guilty.)

Gregg: Well, when you get over this illness we'll have to make up for lost time, eh? (I'm to the point I can't fathom us ever leading a normal life, in the bedroom or elsewhere.)

Sherrie: Hubba hubba. (And what if this illness doesn't go away? Will you go away, Gregg?)

Gregg: Well, get some sleep. (I want some sleep, too. Like Rip Van Winkle. If I'm lucky I'll wake up in 20 years. I'm so damned tired of hearing "no" every night. I'm so damned tired of everything about this life.)

Sherrie: Maybe we can make love tomorrow. (Of course I think all you really want is sex, not love. How could you possibly love a loser like me?)

Gregg: Sure, we'll see. (I know sex is the last thing you want to worry about. How can she really love me if she can't stand the thought of touching me?)

Sherrie: Good night, I love you. (I wish you knew how much I really love you.)

Gregg: Good night, I love you, too. (What the heck am I doing wrong here?)

I know what the heck we were doing wrong back then. We were not putting voice to the parentheses. If you operate primarily in the pseudo-community phase, you believe the unspoken words above should remain mute. They say too much. They put a terrifying emotional spin to a conversation that could easily get out of control. But the spoken words in the dialogue above dim the true messages, cutting off the open and honest communication that could have occurred. Staying in Phase one is akin to having the Broncos and Packers play two-hand-touch instead of bone-crunching-tackle in Super Bowl XXXII. Pseudo-community takes the LIFE out of living.

The spoken words didn't capture the essence of what we were thinking and feeling. They did not provide the springboard to breakthrough conversation – the kind that is memorable and enriching. The words in parentheses – words such as needy, wrapping your arms around me, nightmare, guilty and Rip Van Winkle – could have catapulted our conversation into a higher stratosphere than ever before. As it was, we used the same, tired, polite and constrained words that kept us grounded in our pain and frustration.

In a sense, because we were stuck in the pseudo-community phase, we robbed our relationship of the zest it needed just as much as chronic illness did. Pseudo-community behavior coupled with the trials of chronic illness can kill the relationship with your loved one. After the first few years of Sherrie's illness, phase one and chronic illness had set us up for the kill.

Spiritual:
Ungodly Relationships

— *or* —

Exposing "The Comforter"

You know the type. They descend on loved ones at the funerals of their dearly departed. "We know he (or she) is in a better place now," they say with a toothy grin. "It's truly a blessing that he (or she) went now. Praise be to God." I sarcastically call people who believe they can bring you comfort in time of grief or loss, "the comforter." As they go, "comforters" are extremely uncomfortable with discomfort and often fail to understand that most others see through the phoniness of their silly grins and syrupy words. Most loved ones I know of, in the midst of their sorrow, feel anger toward "the comforter." The loss of a beloved friend or relative changes their lives forever. They feel indescribable pain in a part of their souls they didn't even know existed. And then along comes "the comforter" with the plastered smile and fatuous words, conveying the message that this whole thing is not really a big deal. "The comforter" might just as easily be talking about the issuance of a parking ticket rather than the death of a loved one.

Within the pseudo-community phase, "the comforter" is a model citizen and a blood brother to the "caretaker." "The comforter" unfailingly seeks comfort, wears masks, squashes emotion and avoids the deeper issues presented by a serious issue, even death. He or she believes life is meant to be easy and will even treat the death of loved ones as a minor inconvenience. I don't like "comforters" or their ways.

Let me shift course for a moment. I believe we all have multiple personalities. It's as if a whole group of specialists lives within your body, forming a township that adds up to the total package that is you. Sometimes your creative personality takes center stage. Other times your organizational expert steps to the plate. An author possesses an internal "writer," a creative, stream-of-consciousness sort who dreams about verbs and is often moody. Within that author dwells an internal "editor," a cigar-chomping, hairy-knuckled bully who slashes and burns the overgrown weed patch of words produced by the "writer."

I have several internal personalities available to take center stage at various times of my life. Unfortunately, one of them is my very own "comforter." He pulls the same kind of garbage on me as described above. He tries to belittle problems and my emotional responses to them. Like a carnival huckster, he tries to divert my attention. He takes my focus away from the realities and the emotions of tough issues. He slips rose-colored lenses over my eyes and heart. And in the process of doing all these things, my "comforter" harms my relationship with God.

I believe in a higher power, which I'll call God. Obviously, God can mean many things to many people. Part of my understanding of God is that, indeed, he is literally a "higher" power. When I'm at my lowest, I have the greatest need for help from the highest – God. But my "comforter" plays the role of a sleazy middleman, often preventing me from going to God with my concerns.

I remember thinking in the early days of Sherrie's illness that something tragic was happening. I needed to talk to close friends and connect with my God, but the internal "comforter" often put the kibosh on such discussions and connections. "Hey, Sherrie will get well soon," he would say. "It's not as if she's dying or anything. Besides, why make yourself vulnerable to your buddies. It will just embarrass them and you. And, look, God's got much more important concerns than one woman's health problems. This isn't that big of a deal. Just suck it up, Gregg, and do what you have to do as the good and solid 'caretaker.' By the way, don't be stupid enough to bring up any of your worries to Sherrie. That will just throw her for a loop. You need to comfort her as I comfort you."

My "comforter" whitewashed the reality of my life with a cheap coat of paint. Rather than allowing me to build better relationships with Sherrie, friends and God, he put me in a relational straitjacket. By helping prevent my grief, he also prevented any relational or personal growth in those early years of Sherrie's illness.

When many people hear or read the word "God," they think of religion. And when many people think of religion, they think of rules. To me, the relationships I maintain are more important than rules in my personal religion. That means I want a relationship with this higher power. Going bowling weekly with a friend is one thing. Talking with a buddy about the pain and frustration of life is something entirely different. Going to church weekly is one thing, while seeking the wisdom and love of God through the pain and frustration of life resides on another plane.

Yes, I need comfort in many areas of my life, including the challenge of responding to Sherrie's ongoing illness. I need comfort that is real, not phony. I need comfort that brings growth, not stagnation. And the first step in obtaining this true comfort is to send my internal "comforter" on a long errand after he has stripped the whitewash paint off tough issues. I need to see the issue in all its gory details and let my emotions fly unfettered. I need to know that I need.

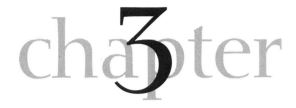

LABELS &
MINDSETS

You will see how "caretakers" and "patients" get boxed in.

Wanted: Superhero

— *or* —

A Formula for Excellence

Wanted: *Someone to assist chronically ill person with demands of life. Must be dependable, caring and organized. In addition, applicant must be creative, humorous and romantic. Willingness to drop everything to assist in crises is a requirement. Applicant must also be a great conversationalist who knows how to have fun. Counseling skills are a major plus. An emphasis on group and family dynamics is desirable. Prefer Jungian to Freudian school of thought. Advanced first-aid certification is a plus. Must be good with kids, know how to prepare a decent meal, have exceptional housecleaning skills and be great (yet sensitive) in bed. Since this is a part-time job, applicant must also hold down a full-time job. Apply only if willing to make a lifelong commitment.*

The "caretaker" paradox is that sometimes we feel as if we must be the superhero described above. These job requirements are unrealistic and unhealthy. Seeking excellence is cool and healthy. Seeking perfection is a stress-producing drag. Many "caretakers" keep their mouths shut and emotions stymied as they march down the perilous path toward perfection. It's a tough – no, impossible – trek to make, especially when it feels as if the whole weight of a family or friendship depends on doing everything without error. Oh, the noble attempt at perfection looks and sounds as if it's the right thing to do. This is especially true because of all the kudos the "perfect caretaker" receives from the outside world. However, people who attempt to fulfill the job description do a grave disservice to themselves and their significant others.

The successful applicant above would have to be a competent friend, homemaker, counselor, spouse, daycare specialist and lover, among other things. Each of those labels comes with a whole list of perceived or required skills and duties. I got in trouble when I tried to play all the roles at one time. I became unhealthy myself. I wore out my brain, my body and my spirit. I went through the duties of each day carrying a figurative 100-pound weight. My body would periodically shut down. "Hey, Gregg," my body would say, "you refuse to take my advice so I'm going to force you to take a time out." Wham! I was hit with the 72-hour flu. If sickness didn't get me, exhaustion or malaise did. A good chunk of the 1980s is as memorable and remarkable as a bad two-hour lecture on a hot summer afternoon.

So how do we overcome this "caretaker" paradox of trying to do too much? One way to address the issue is to delegate. Most successful business leaders understand the power of delegation. We can apply those skills to helping a loved one who is sick. After several years of trying to achieve the impossible, I chose a healthier approach to how I support Sherrie. Instead of fulfilling that avalanche of job responsibilities, I elected to focus my energies on loving Sherrie. Repeat: Loving Sherrie. Note that I used a verb (loving) rather than a noun (such as the labels lover or spouse) to describe my focus. Labels bring responsibilities, while loving involves activities. Responsibilities are specific and confining, whereas loving provides endless possibilities mixed with doses of exhilaration.

By seeking to love Sherrie I could surrender the onerous task of being "the friend" or "the counselor." I could be a friend and an occasional amateur counselor, but other people could provide friendship and counseling as well. Both Sherrie and I do better when we have a friend or two with whom to talk and have fun. I didn't always feel that way. As a young husband, I convinced myself that I was all Sherrie needed for companionship. As I grew more wise and mature I realized that school of thought was a crock of you-know-what. A self-confident person knows he or she does not have to be the only friend in town for someone who is close to you.

For example, my "friendliness" is different from the "friendliness" Sherrie shares with her close acquaintance Diana. Sometimes a 30-minute walk with Diana is just what the doctor ordered for Sherrie. I just might not feel like going on a walk that day or I might go, but be angry because I felt coerced. It would be yet another duty to perform. Diana loves to walk around Lake Loveland with close friends. While Sherrie and Diana circle the lake, I can do something I need to do for work or as a parent or, believe it or not, for myself.

I believe in counseling and consider people who go to counselors as being more healthy and courageous than those who don't. A good counselor is more than a good conversationalist who knows how to ask open-ended questions and practice active listening. I can and do those things with Sherrie often. Yet, there is another huge role counselors play that I can't. You wouldn't want a nonprofessional friend to perform minor surgery on your body. Likewise, you are playing with matches if a nonprofessional friend (or lover or spouse) practices in-depth counseling and advice. I recommend you pay for a counselor's unbiased professional services if you can afford it. Many companies now have Employee Assistance Programs (EAP) that provide low-cost counseling for employees and their dependents.

You can also delegate some household duties. The kids will balk at first, but getting them more involved might make them feel better about themselves – especially because you NEED them to help you out. We all want to feel needed. And if finances allow it, having someone come weekly to spruce up the place can be money well spent.

A person who is chronically ill probably does need a lover, a significant other, a counselor, a buddy, a maid and all the rest. In our case, I lay sole claim as Sherrie's lover and significant other. But I share or delegate the responsibilities for many of those other roles. Focus on loving your loved one rather than performing duties for your "patient." It will be easier on you and more helpful for the person who is ill. It also allows other key people to feel the joy of helping. Replace the cumbersome garbage of the superhero job description with this memorable equation:

Love + Delegation = Support Excellence

The Foul Cloak of Guilt

— *or* —

Tell Them to "Take a Hike"

We didn't have enough money for a vacation in 1995, so Sherrie felt guilty. "If we didn't have such high medical expenses we would have enough money for everything we need and want." she said. She is right, I told myself, then I felt guilty for silently agreeing. I headed to New England for four days to run a training seminar. We needed the money, you know. But I felt guilty leaving Sherrie alone with a migraine headache, neck pain and three strong-willed children. Sherrie felt guilty about being angry about my business trip. A month later Sherrie went in for a neck fusion and felt guilty about throwing our family's life for a loop again. And as nurses wheeled her away to the operating room, I felt guilty about being the one who sat in the waiting room while she faced the knife.

Sometimes we miraculously overcome our guilt but get busted by the Guilt Police. We are our own worst critics, but there are plenty of other able-bodied, feeble-minded folks out there who inject strong doses of guilt if we let down our guards. In the January-February 1994 issue of *Arthritis Today* magazine, I wrote an article about the need to grieve over Sherrie's chronic illness. I included my feelings and thoughts that described living with someone who is ill. In the following issue of the magazine, four readers wrote letters to the editor in response to my article. Vivien of Stony Brook, N.Y., wrote:

"Not once in Gregg Piburn's diatribe did he say anything about getting his wife into a support group. Only that he cleans the house and takes care of the kids and rushes his wife to the emergency room. I agree, being a caretaker is a wearying and often thankless ordeal, but has it ever occurred to Mr. Piburn that his wife also needs strong emotional support to deal with her infirmities? No matter how bad things get, he at least has the option of getting away for a while."

Vivien failed to understand that the article was about me, not Sherrie. She assumed that, because I did not mention support groups and emotional support, I obviously provided neither for Sherrie. She could not handle an article that did not focus on the sick person and the illness. She decided to publicly dump a crap-load of guilt on me for having the gall to share my struggles and feelings.

Not surprisingly, part of me wondered if she made the correct assessment. That's right, I felt a tinge of guilt. The three other letters however, were extremely positive.

Fran of Herrick Center, Pa., wrote, "Reading 'Breaking the Grief Barrier' (the title of my article) and the other letters and articles on fibromyalgia has saved me and given me hope." Penny of Rocklin, Calif., wrote, "Gregg Piburn's story touched the emotional side of so many family members, the grief they must endure and the special problems unique to their situation." And Diana of Dunbar, W.V. wrote: "'Breaking the Grief Barrier' . . . was both touching and insightful. The way he described how his life had changed since his wife developed fibromyalgia was very informative to me as a victim of this syndrome."

Sometimes I fall back into the label of "caretaker" and feel guilty about writing that article and this book. Gosh, I say, dumbfounded, am I coming across as a victim? Did Vivien hit the nail on the head? Interestingly, I forget the three positive letters and focus only on Vivien's. I become a sponge in search of guilt, an activity that depresses and soils the soul.

I left a cozy corporate job in 1991 to start a one-person consulting business. "You are crazy," said a former co-worker who dedicates his life to comfort, planning and predictability. I could easily live with such a bland person calling me crazy. However, I read into his numerous comments that I was crazy AND selfish. I told him I had longed for years to be my own boss. I finally had a chance to make this lifelong dream a reality but, as my friend pointed out, the seed of that dream came to life before chronic illness put a whammy on Sherrie. I not only had to wrestle with whether I could achieve business success on my own, I also had to overcome strong feelings of guilt.

Author Anthony de Mello said: "In life, one plays the hand one is dealt to the best of one's ability. Those who insist on playing not the hand they were given, but the one they insist they should have been dealt, these are life's failures. We are not asked if we will play; that is not an option. Play we must; the option is how."

Sherrie did not maliciously choose to become chronically ill. I did not decide to remain physically healthy to spite her. Fate dealt Sherrie and I the hand that led to our current situation. For numerous reasons, this hand called chronic illness comes loaded with wild cards called guilt. Neither of us need feel guilty.

What we do need however, is to determine how we play this hand. And dealing with chronic illness while wearing foul cloaks of guilt will only exacerbate an already difficult situation. In general, those who live with people who have ongoing illness are just too nice and polite. That's part of our job description. Here is something we can do, though, to rid ourselves of that vile cloak. We can tell Vivien and all the other Guilt Cops to take a hike. And then . . . and then, my friends, we must not feel guilty about it.

Dysfunctional Doctors

— *or* —

Forming a Great Medical Team

Doctors are not deities. Some doctors are dysfunctional. Do not depend on diagnoses developed in the dark. For two years I helped facilitate a two-day course titled, "Baseline Training," which helped community members better understand addiction and family dysfunction. I believe all families are dysfunctional to some degree. The more dysfunctional a family, the more clear-cut individuals' roles are within the family.

For example, in a classic alcoholic home with both dependent and co-dependent parents, children tend to play distinct roles. Such a family will have children who, in dysfunctional-family vernacular, each play one of four roles: hero, scapegoat, lost child or mascot. The dynamics of extreme dysfunction lead individuals to play these narrowly defined roles as a way for the family to survive within its unhealthy state. I've found that the pseudo-community phase is another brand of dysfunction, although in a more subtle form than a family in crisis. In phase one, people also play clearly defined roles.

Within a pseudo-community work group, managers often have a monopoly on answers. Employees in such a group might see a problem and have an easy answer, but will simply wait for a manager to step forward and give the "official" answer. In such a group, it might be perfectly all right for

Eddie (the group "mascot") to play a practical joke at a staff meeting. However, if Vince (the group "scapegoat") pulls the same stunt, the boss will publicly criticize him.

So what does this have to do with chronic illness? The "patient," "caretaker" and medical staff (doctors, specialists, nurses) form a team. Such a group often falls into the realm of the pseudo-community. And if nothing else, groups that display the behavior characteristics of the pseudo-community phase are dishonest and ineffective. In the pseudo-community, the doctor or specialist is the boss who has the responsibility to fix the illness. Everyone expects these experts to have all the answers. Their intense and lengthy training points them down that narrow path.

In Sherrie's case, answers were hard to find. The mysterious nature of fibromyalgia stumped many doctors, especially early on in our search for a diagnosis. This frustrated everyone involved, sometimes the doctors as much as Sherrie and me. Clear-cut answers failed to materialize . . . so some doctors made up other "answers" (read: guesses, to be more accurate), because that was their role. Remember, people who are in the pseudo-community phase expect life to be easy. They hate to struggle with difficult problems involving hard-to-find solutions. Unfortunately, we sought assistance from some doctors who would rather give easy, pat answers than conduct research on what Sherrie's symptoms might indicate. They preferred stating their guesses as solutions, rather than admitting they were baffled.

Sherrie – who hates to operate within the narrow parameters of phase one – was unafraid to tell doctors that a previous diagnosis and action plan seemed off base. "I tried it, but felt worse than before," she would say calmly and honestly.

Some doctors could not handle a patient taking such an active role in problem solving. Those doctors tended to say at that point things such as:

- "Well, you'll just have to give it more time to work."
- "I doubt if you really followed the program thoroughly."
- "I think you're just having a bad day today. It's really working."
- "Well, if that's not working all I can assume is maybe the problem is more mental than physical."

All of those responses illustrate a phase-one mentality. Without using these exact words, they convey the following messages.

- I'm the boss.
- I have a monopoly on answers.
- You are stepping on my turf.
- The problem can't be that difficult.
- Trust me, because I know best.
- If I can't do my job it's because you are screwing up the process.

How do you combat falling into pseudo-community mode within the medical maze? Unfortunately, it might be impossible to break out of that treacherous phase if the doctor revels in his or her know-it-all role. I'll be the first to admit that if the know-it-all doc really does know it all, then it might, MIGHT, be worth being treated as a second-class citizen who should only speak when spoken to. Personally, a doctor would have to be the Michael Jordan of physicians for me to withstand second-class citizenship.

Before walking out on any doctor, however, the "caretaker" and/or "patient" must clearly state how you hope the group can work as a team. Tell the doctor that you need everyone involved to be open and honest in diagnosing and treating the specific condition. Ask many questions and provide thorough and accurate information about how the ill person feels now and between appointments. Open communication figuratively "turns on the light" as the group seeks answers and solutions. If you try open communication and you still hit a brick wall, then seek a more open and progressive doctor.

Don't get the idea I hate the whole medical establishment. Indeed, I don't. We have met many skilled, honest and personable doctors and specialists on the long trail of Sherrie's illness. Medical professionals have helped Sherrie through horrendous physical struggles. A few key doctors and specialists have been alongside her for much of the journey on the road to overall improvement. But our paths have crossed with a few who did more harm than good in subtle and not-so-subtle ways.

You lose some degree of control in your life when chronic illness intrudes. Don't give up all control as you deal with doctors and specialists. Insist on open and honest communication as the team searches for medical answers. Don't be afraid to tell a doctor that something is not working. Tell the doctor you expect him or her to admit when the illness stumps them rather than pretending they know the answer.

The good news is there are doctors and specialists who welcome such partnership with those who are ill and the people who love them. They are not afraid to seek the expertise of other professionals in the search for solutions. True, doctors are not deities, but there are many who function effectively and will work with you to discover the real causes of your loved one's symptoms.

The Fragile China Doll

— or —

Robbed of Life

You walk through the expensive gift shop and your eyes lock on a gorgeous and fragile china doll. You reach for your wallet and moments later carefully walk the wrapped china doll to your car. When you get home, the first thing you do is unwrap the precious new possession and place it on the mantelpiece.

I was going crazy in a corporate job that put me in a warm and soft straitjacket. I thought I might go crazy if I spent another year, month, hour or minute there. I considered telling Sherrie about my frustration, but she had more pressing problems to consider than my silly little career. But, damn, I thought I might snap one day. I again considered telling her. No, my job was to protect her from emotional issues, not bring them up. I had to provide comfort, not discomfort.

The china doll exists in an enchanted atmosphere out of the reach of wiggling nephews and wagging dog tails. You protect it like an endangered species. It is a privileged possession perched high above the maddening crowd.

"I'm home, Dad," said our oldest daughter, Corlet. "Where's Mom? I need to tell her something important."

"No, no, no. Don't go in there. She's resting. What do you need?"

"I need to talk to Mom."

"Well, let me help you."

"No, I need Mom."

"Listen, we can't wake her up. Just let me help you."

"But I want Mom."

"You can't have her now. She needs her rest. Can it wait till later?"

"No, I'll just forget it."

Sometimes china dolls come to life as someone who is chronically ill. Their loved ones become the person who protects that fragile doll.

"I got the part!" Sherrie said.

"Oh, the role in the community play?"

"Yeah, I can't believe they chose me."

"Well, I hope it doesn't take too much out of you."

"You seem worried about me."

"How many nights a week will you rehearse?"

"Five nights a week for six weeks."

"Whew, that's a lot."

"You're right. Am I crazy to do this?"

"Well, it's your decision, but . . ."

"I am crazy aren't I?"

"No, but you do have to take care of yourself."

"Hmm, maybe I better call now so they can get someone to replace me before rehearsals begin."

For several years I treated Sherrie like a china doll. I became the buffer between her and the real life of teacher conferences and bills, parties and conflicts, appointments and truth. That last item is the most important. I kept my china doll from the truth for fear it would bog her down rather than set her free.

"No, I'll go to Alyse's awards banquet," I said moments after walking in the door after work.

"But you must be beat, Gregg," Sherrie said.

"No, I'm fine."

"But I really want to go. Also, I think Alyse would like me to be there."

"I know you want to go and I know Alyse would like you there. But you were busy this morning and have two doctor appointments tomorrow. You have to pace yourself."

"Well, I feel tired. But you look exhausted yourself."

"I'm fine. Just let me go. You can 'veg' in front of the TV."

"OK."

Imagine finding out as a young adult that your father didn't die in the war but split from the family long ago in the cover of night. Or imagine being a woman whose elderly mother refuses to tell you about her terminal disease until mere days before death. You look back and realize you had been operating in the dark. People had failed to enlighten you on important matters. You feel cheated by people who hide the truth. You feel like a china doll, stuck on a mantelpiece, above that nasty, dirty, energizing, wondrous, it's-all-we've-got-thing called life.

"Gregg, are you sure you're being honest with us?" the counselor said. "Now would be a perfect time to tell how you really feel about Sherrie's latest health setback."

"Yeah, I'm being honest. As I said, I'm disappointed but I know we can make it through this just as we have made it through the last several years."

"But Gregg," Sherrie said, "I really want to hear what's in your heart, not just what's on your mind."

"I'm telling you two, I'm dis-a-poin-ted. What else do you want from me?"

"I just sense you're holding back some, Gregg," the counselor said. "I think it would help you and I know it would help Sherrie if you were totally truthful with us."

"Are you calling me a liar?"

"No, but . . ."

"Geez, I feel like a prisoner of war here. I'm disappointed. That's it. We move on."

"Ohh-kay," the counselor said.

Sherrie stares out the window and says nothing.

Chronic illness robs a person of many aspects of life. By treating Sherrie like a china doll I took even more of life away from her. Sometimes friends vanish, jobs end, vacations become extinct and goals fade away because of illness. As if that was not loss enough, we can strip the last semblance of humanity away by putting our loved ones on a figurative mantelpiece.

"Is everything OK, Gregg?"

"Yeah, Sherrie, everything's fine."

"Are you sure?"

"Yep."

China dolls might be treated like mantelpiece ornaments but they know when they're being given a line.

I took Sherrie off the mantelpiece and now – even when she's physically down – I see her break through the porcelain veneer and relish the humanity of life.

As usual, I waited until the last minute to get my 1997 income tax figures together for my accountant. I realized my schedule prevented me from completing the task unless I pulled a couple of all-nighters. Then I got a brilliant idea. I asked for Sherrie's help.

"Really?" she said, putting down a blanket she'd been quilting for a soon-to-be-born niece or nephew. "I like doing that kind of stuff." I quickly handed her check registers, notebook paper and a calculator. Getting figures together for income tax is not typically considered a fun activity. But it felt good to Sherrie because it was real life performed by a real person.

A Daydreaming Indiana Jones

— *or* —

The Family "Jug of Wine"

One of the labels I coveted in the 1980s was "family leader." Many of the books I read and tapes I listened to challenged men to become strong family leaders. As with all labels, this one came with a whole set of preconceived responsibilities and goals – not all necessarily good. Yet, in many ways my personality failed to match those expectations of a family leader – which isn't necessarily all bad. In truth, Sherrie had always been the true family leader. For example, she made most of the important decisions during the first 12 years of our marriage.

For the first 35 years of my life, I earned a doctorate in daydreaming. I was to daydreaming what Bill Cosby is to comedy. I was a high-school jock and big-time dreamer who assumed I would become a professional athlete. I devised a baseball game played with a deck of cards and fabricated my Major League career with pages of statistics documenting my success. While young Mike Schmidts and Dave Winfields played ball year-round, honing skills required to make "the Show" (the big leagues), I fiddled away my days, expecting dreams to turn true, producing a long-running show of my own that was pure fiction and false prophecy.

When chronic illness walloped her, Sherrie started struggling with what brand of bread to buy, what color sweater to wear; forget the big decisions. Uh-oh. Ship without a captain.

For years friction existed between the part of me that sought adventure and the part that demanded security. I was the reckless Indiana Jones teamed with the corporate accountant. The internal numbers guy always won out, causing relief mixed with a dose of self-hatred.

When Sherrie and I had to cancel our Mexico City trip in 1985, relief overruled disappointment in my brain. This time the fearful internal accountant had not crushed my daydream. Adventure is not an option when your wife can barely make it to the grocery store. Sherrie's new illness allowed me to imagine wondrous experiences without the angst of deciding whether to take a bold step. Chronic illness was the perfect out for me – I didn't have to back up my dreams with action and people began giving me four-star ratings as a family leader. Indiana Jones and the corporate accountant both got what they wanted.

For months at a time in the late 1980s Sherrie retreated to the bedroom or sat in front of the television, too weary or sad to face people or projects. Sherrie's illness forced me to spend more time with the kids, do more housework and make more decisions. To my surprise and delight, kudos came pouring in from admirers.

"Gregg, you are a rock."

"What would Sherrie do without you?"

"I couldn't handle this as well as you do."

"Sherrie is so lucky having you stand by her."

These comments boosted my ego, made me feel like a family leader, told me I was living up to that label. For the first time in our marriage, I felt as if I was truly meeting my obligations and it felt good.

Damn, did you grasp what I just said? As Sherrie felt worse, I felt better. That is horse shit! That is the mark of a person sick in the head. It also represents a win/lose philosophy. For someone to be a winner, somebody else has to be a loser. By some mysterious flip of a coin, Sherrie, not I, became chronically ill. She lost and I won.

Family members in the quintessential alcoholic home play out the following scene. The husband gets blitzed on Sunday and suffers from a hangover on Monday. The co-dependent wife calls the office to say her husband has the flu and won't be in today. Her actions help allow the disease to keep its stranglehold on the family.

Periodically, the wife thinks about leaving her husband for good. But what would she do? What role would she play in this crazy drama called life? She has a role as a co-dependent spouse in an alcoholic family. The family as they know it would crumble if she failed to play her role.

Let's say that her husband chooses to turn and face the enemy, the bottle, eyeball-to-eyeball. Perhaps he goes through a 12-step program and becomes a recovering alcoholic. He refrains from the bottle and never misses another day of work.

That's great news for the wife, right? In the long run, we expect that to be true. But during the initial transitional phase it might not be great news at all for the wife. The husband and the family system no longer need the duties she performed. Before, her actions brought meaning and shaky stability to the family. Now those actions are unnecessary and she feels useless.

I became dependent on Sherrie's illness for my egotistical kicks, making me the co-dependent in our family structure. Her illness gave me new meaning in life. At long last, I had climbed the ladder to that family-leader rung, gaining the admiration of friends and acquaintances. Periodically, Sherrie would go through a month or two when she felt halfway decent. During those times I would subconsciously find ways to throw tension into the equation, spoiling what could have been wonderful times of respite or pure fun. That was when I said I wanted to leave my secure job or move to Montana.

Of course, I knew I would not have to follow through on those pipe dreams. Sherrie was not so sure whether I would take those bold steps. Being in the pseudo-community phase, I certainly kept her in the dark regarding my true intentions. Then, her symptoms would flare up again and I could go back to my "caretaker" duties, which I hated and loved simultaneously. Sherrie's illness was the family's jug of wine and I was the family's sick pseudo-leader.

(*note*
The dynamics of addiction and whether the wife should leave are complex issues without easy answers. I suggest you read *Co-dependent No More* by Melody Beattie for insight into those issues.)

Section One Action Page:
Break Out of the Box

NOTE: I suggest you buy a notebook to use in conjunction with this book and its action pages. To get the most out of this book, be sure to work on these action pages. They will greatly improve your odds of getting the best out of the book. Write answers to the action page assignments in the book or in a notebook.

1. Make a job description

Take a sheet of paper and describe your role as a "caretaker." Include in your job description the duties you perform and the personality traits that personify someone fulfilling that role. For example:

DUTIES	PERSONALITY TRAITS
• Provide child care after school	• Accept "assignments" with a smile
• Protect "patient" from nuisances	• Selectively dishonest
• _____	• _____
• _____	• _____
• _____	• _____
• _____	• _____

and so on . . .

(NOTE: If you are chronically ill, do Numbers 1 and 2 from the "patient" perspective.)

2. Assess your job description

• Which of the duties and personality traits, when viewed rationally, seem erroneous?

• How are these erroneous duties and traits impacting the "patient," your relationship with the "patient," and you?

• How could you change these duties and traits in a way that would be more helpful and healthy for the "patient," the relationship and you?

3. Consider the china doll

In what ways are you treating a person who is chronically ill as you would a china doll? Write down your thoughts and feelings about this topic. After reading this entire book and getting insight on how to approach such a conversation, consider talking about the key points with the person who is chronically ill.

4. Mine for gold

• Out of all the essays and suggested activities in this section, which one do you believe provides the most significant and/or memorable nugget of information for you?

_____

_____

_____

• What is the "first step" you will take toward making that nugget truly impact your life for the better?

- I will _____
  _____what?)
by _____
  _____(when?)

EXAMPLE: I will help my significant other prepare for an upcoming doctor's appointment and I will accompany her to that appointment within the next three weeks.

THE WORLD GOES KABLOOEY!

(**Chaos.** Populated by angry people. Epitomized by anger, back biting, win–lose thinking.)

phase two

"*It's me against the world.*"

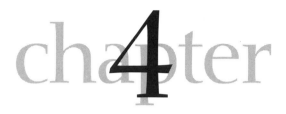

SOMETHING
SNAPS

Even though chaotic behavior seems shocking to pseudo-community residents, it can be a step in the right direction. See how you can enter the phase of chaos without destroying your relationship with your chronically ill loved one and family.

Red Streaks on Gray Day

— *or* —

Father Shows Worst

The day outside seemed as lifeless and colorless as an industry-standard metal desk. My insides felt just as dull and heavy. However, I was not in a corporate cubicle, having escaped that environment 14 months before. But my spirit still felt as small and cramped as an 8-foot-by-8-foot office cube. On that gray December day in 1992, I worked on a freelance writing project – at home – which the Eisenhower years of my childhood had taught me was to be a man's castle, the place he returned to at the end of a long day's battle on the job. Home was the place where loved ones await each man as he looks forward to an evening of warm fellowship and mellow respite.

I know such a view of home life seems anachronistic in contemporary times. Being a "man of the '90s," I feel embarrassed to admit that a part of me wished for gentle evenings of "Father-Knows-Best" splendor within a mythical stronghold in the suburbs.

It's not surprising I longed for an unrealistic haven. Sherrie had been in the hospital during the Christmas season, which thrust our family into a tailspin. While Sherrie struggled with back pain and other health-related issues, I struggled miserably to keep my consulting business afloat while also keeping track of three strong-willed children who missed their mom.

To make matters worse, an invisible chasm separated Sherrie and me. That December we had reached the low point of our relationship.

One afternoon not long after recovering from her stint in hospital, Sherrie took Alyse on an errand. That left me with Corlet and Bret. I shut down my computer because I knew their demands would sap my creative juices for the rest of the day.

Corlet and Bret went to separate parts of the house and I trudged to the kitchen to wash a big stack of dirty dishes – the perfect activity to match my mood. Every time I walked between the kitchen and my home office I stepped over magazines I assumed Corlet had scattered at the top of the stairs the previous night.

"Hey, Corlet," I said, "please come pick up these magazines." She came into the kitchen and claimed she picked them up before school and somebody else had strewn them onto the floor. "It's not my job," she said with the inflection of a workplace troublemaker. She walked to the kitchen table and sat down, opening a book to read.

"Corlet," I said while standing by the sink, "I need your help, so please do it for me." She continued to read, acting as if I were a gnat whose buzz wasn't quite discernible.

All of a sudden the gnat – me – turned into a giant, angry hornet. I spun my whole body around and purposely knocked the packed dish drainer off the counter. A glass baking pan went kablooey on the floor as I screamed a guttural sound devoid of words. I kicked a large plastic bowl down the stairs and yelled about how nobody gave me any respect. Corlet looked at her Rodney-Dangerfield dad from the top of the stairs, while Bret looked shocked from the bottom of the steps.

"I can't stand being treated like this!" I yelled.

I walked past Bret and out the front door. Corlet got to the door just as it slammed behind me. She opened it and said with a hint of desperation, "Don't go."

I turned and, with the histrionic fury of a high-school drama student, told my 11-year-old daughter, "I'm going for a walk . . . and I may or may not come back." I marched down the street like a brazen soldier heading to the battlefield. Behind me I heard Corlet say: "Come on, Dad. I'm sorry. Please come back." I refused to look back as my feet continued to thud down the sidewalk.

Emotional abuse is an ugly thing. For the next 10 minutes I walked. I'm not sure if the noise was fact or fiction, but in the distance I heard a child scream. Was it one of my children yelling for a lost dad? I hoped it was not, but felt too disoriented and ashamed to rush home to find out. For a minute I considered what our lives would be like if I vanished forever. The shocking answer that came to mind was that everyone's life might be better. But I couldn't just walk out on the family – especially on those two kids who seemed distraught when I left.

I returned home and found a note on the front door. It read: "Dad, Mom & Alyse: Me and Bret went to look for Dad on my bike and the trailer. Corlet. ps: Dad, I'm sorry." Corlet refused to pick up a few magazines so now she and her 4-year-old brother searched the neighborhood for their disillusioned and disappointing dad. In this instance of grief and angst I had become an emotional adolescent trying to parent three kids.

I sat on the porch and waited, too exhausted to begin a counter-search. Five minutes later I saw Corlet chugging down the street on her bike. She looked worn out – a foreign expression for one so strong willed. Bret, sitting inside the trailer compartment, looked content, as if he viewed the whole episode as an exciting game of "Hunt For The Missing Dad."

One thing I've learned as a parent is the power of the words "I'm sorry." I apologized to both of them separately. With my 11-year-old daughter, I could be more expansive in my apology. I told her how angry, confused and stressed I felt with everything going on in our lives. I told her how much I missed Sherrie when she was away. Corlet understood everything I said because she felt many of the same emotions.

"You know," I said with my arm around Corlet, "I would never hit you or do terrible things physically to you, don't you?" She looked at me with a face more innocent than expected for a child growing up in my home. She replied, "Anybody who knows you knows that would never happen." Those were powerful and comforting words coming from a beloved child.

Moving from the comfort of the pseudo-community phase to the discomfort of the chaos phase can be shocking. I do not condone emotional abuse, which is how I classify my actions that gray day in 1992. By the time you finish section two, you will understand that there are other ways to venture into phase two without making an emotional outburst or intensifying a situation to the point of crisis.

This might be hard to understand, considering my inability to contain my anger, but I contend that generally it is the pseudo-community phase rather than the chaos phase that is the most harmful to a family, especially one trying to stay afloat in the midst of chronic illness. Without discomfort there is no personal growth. Without moving to phase two there is little meaningful communication. The grayness of the pseudo-community phase is transformed to a phase-two picture streaked with jagged lightning bolts of red, representing the anger that comes out in chaos. Anger, folks, is not bad; it just is. What's important is how you respond to anger.

People impacted directly or indirectly by chronic illness can't help feeling angry. In the long run, it is more healthy to bring that anger to the fore instead of keeping it locked up inside. And if you can release that anger in more small, frequent outbursts you can decrease the chances of it exploding in ways that might damage loved ones and relationships irrevocably.

By always playing the "caretaker" role, I had held my anger in too long and when I let it go, it resulted in a hideous tantrum.

More than five years have passed since that bleak episode. On this brilliant March day in 1998, while writing this essay, I see Corlet walk in from school. I go up to my 17-year-old daughter who already has the cordless phone propped on her shoulder as she talks to a friend. I put my arm around her. "Just a second," she says into the phone. "Why did you do that?" she says suspiciously. "Oh, I just missed you today. I'm glad you're home." Before she goes back to her phone friend, she flashes a glorious smile and says, "Thanks."

Growing Thick & Gnarled

— *or* —

Tutu Reminders

I wore a tutu on my job. No, I'm not a ballerina and I only did it once on the time clock. Not surprisingly, a corporate videographer captured my performance for posterity. I'm not proud that certain evil co-workers sometimes show my ballerina impersonation to laughing groups of corporate managers and employees. But even such a silly thing as businessmen making fools of themselves provided an important reminder for me today.

Thirteen years ago, myself and three colleagues performed a strange ballet to the tune of a country and western song as part of a United Way celebration. Ron, one of the "dancers," retired today after a 32-year career and 60 of his co-workers attended a farewell luncheon. I still do some consulting for my old firm, so Ron's manager invited me to attend the celebration. Someone pulled the video out of mothballs and showed it to the group, all of whom found the footage hilarious.

I laughed, too, but with a sensitive eye I also zoomed in on that younger version of myself. For one thing, I noticed I looked much different from the person I see when I get out of the shower to dry myself these days. I remembered myself being skinny, but I looked lithe and healthy – which is definitely an advantage for ballerinas of any ilk. I also looked carefree, which is how I was viewed by my co-workers back then.

We performed that pseudo-ballet dance just a few months after Sherrie first got sick. I looked across the 13 years at the young dancer, the younger me, as if I was an elder mentor. I felt extreme sorrow for the young Piburn. He didn't have a clue about the staying power of Sherrie's illness. He did not know what was in store for him and the people he loves most. I saw a dancer who had glided through a relatively easy life. Now, with the wisdom of time on my side, I knew storm clouds had already formed on the horizon of the dancer's life even as he did mock pirouettes. Hell, if I had looked in a crystal ball that afternoon long ago, I might have done anything – sold my soul or sworn to wear a tutu for the next 13 years – to change the forecast of my life with Sherrie. That seems shortsighted now because it supports my early-life belief that life is easy, not difficult. In reality, if it had not been chronic illness, some other difficulty would have stepped forward to offer the many challenges, grief and growth I needed to become the man I am today. Perhaps the real change I would have made is for me to be sick or to at least share in the pain of my wife's ailments. Then again, if I'm totally honest, I would hate to trade my health for Sherrie's.

One of my favorite authors is Alan Jones, an Episcopalian priest who lives and works in San Francisco. In one of his books titled, *The Soul's Journey: Exploring the Three Passages of the Spiritual Life with Dante as a Guide* he wrote the following words: "Marriage has been by far the most powerful text in my life: a spiritual roller coaster of crashes, disasters, and hurts, but also of rescue, forgiveness, and healing – a wondrous garden of renewal." The chaos phase often includes disasters and hurts. We forget it might also bring growth and renewal.

If you live in a family affected by chronic illness, you can surely relate to the first part of Jones's roller coaster with its crashes, disasters and hurts. For me, the roller coaster image brings to mind canceled trips and tight budgets and smelly recovery rooms. The carefree corporate ballerina and his loved ones were about to take many nasty spills.

So yeah, this afternoon I saw a younger and thinner version of myself before "the fall." But when I think back to that younger me, I don't think of rescue or forgiveness or healing. I did not feel the need for renewal. Those were at best vague concepts in the head of that tutu dude.

I have a confession to make. The United Way celebration did not represent my tutu debut. Seven years earlier, before illness and kids, Sherrie and I performed our own funky version of "Sugar Plum Fairies" at a Christmas party for news room employees. Journalists tend to be crazy and my co-workers and I fit the mold. So did our significant others. Sherrie and I had a ball performing to the cacophony of laughter and catcalls in that news room Amateur Hour.

When I recall that night I remember Sherrie and me jumping and twirling, sliding and falling. We were still young lovers with strong and limber bodies. Our relationship did not know crashes, disasters and hurts, nor did it know rescue, forgiveness and healing. The Gregg Piburn who wore tutus looked good, but his heart and soul were as flimsy as a slice of balsa wood. I suppose there is an appropriate season in life when it is fine to prance around in figurative tutus. But chronic illness forced Sherrie and me to move on, to see life from a different perspective, to discover the deeper meaning why we are here. Crashes, disasters, hurts, rescue, forgiveness and healing have nourished and renewed my heart and soul. The balsa wood has grown more thick and gnarled, able to withstand the storms, able to see something good come out of chaos.

Support Group Myths & Tips

— or —

Seeking Solutions, Fellowship & Hope

What can my significant other and I do to get through this ordeal? One answer that may come to mind: "Join a support group." It might be the right answer for you and/or your significant other. But for me this solution closed the door on other options that later proved to be more helpful. When dealing with tough and complex issues such as chronic illness, easy answers aren't usually sufficient.

Sherrie asked me to attend a monthly CFS support group in Denver several years ago. It was a large gathering at which a hefty amount of medical information was presented. Part of each structured meeting included time for members to give updates on their health. A few other spouses and partners, such as myself, sat quietly listening. I figured I was doing my support-group job by being nothing more than Sherrie's trusted and mute sidekick. The way group leaders ignored me supported that thought.

On the drive home, after our fifth meeting, Sherrie said, "You know, I really feel bummed out every time I leave these meetings." Staying with that vernacular, chronic illness is a big enough downer without dumping more of a negative load on a person's psyche. We chose to leave that group and have been selective in our attendance at other support groups.

Here are some support-group "myths" and suggestions from my experience; your experience may be different.

Myth #1: Support-group "customers" are those people who are sick.

In this arrangement, "caretakers" are second-class citizens who are only there to support their ill significant others. In some support groups "caretakers" are treated as if they are invisible. They rarely, if ever, are invited to speak. They might get an occasional pat on the back for "being there" for their significant other, but they definitely have nothing significant to give to or receive from the sessions.

Suggestion #1: Expand the group's mission to include support for "caretakers."

Every time I have spoken at a support group, the members have been pleasantly surprised to have me, rather than Sherrie, speak to the group. Ask support group leaders to consider bringing in literature or speakers to address the challenges of being the person who supports their significant others. If the group won't budge on this request, consider finding a more open-minded group. Another option is for the "patient" to continue attending while the "caretaker" recharges his or her batteries in another way.

Myth #2: The more information you have about the illness, the better off you will be.

Most support groups provide a rich flow of medical information to its members. They often bring in doctors and specialists to speak about the latest findings. Unfortunately, these medical professionals often lack good communication skills or the meeting environment and schedule decreases the chance of an effective flow of information. When I have attended such meetings, I left feeling overloaded with depressing information, not enlightened.

Suggestion #2: Seek a few key nuggets of information.

Be selective about which sessions you attend. You might be in a group that pressures you to attend every session. The last thing individuals or couples need when dealing with chronic illness is another "should" on their regular to-do list. Have the courage to follow your instincts rather than succumbing to the demands of the group. When the group plans a session around a topic of interest, go into the meeting with a few key questions you want answered. Don't try to grasp everything as if the speaker were a college professor who will test you on the material later. Seek answers to your key questions and if you don't find them during the presentation, ask the speaker during a formal question-and-answer period, or on your own, before the person leaves.

Myth #3: There is strength in numbers.

True, there can be value in hearing about the struggles and solutions of others. If nothing else, there is some comfort in finding out you are not alone in battling the vagaries of chronic illness. The fallacy of Myth #3 however, is that numbers alone cannot guarantee personal growth or satisfaction. There is weakness in numbers if the individuals bring you down, and if the group consists of people who irritate or anger you.

Suggestion #3: Find a group of open and honest people you like.

Finding fellowship in a support group is at least as important as finding facts about your loved one's illness. Remember that most groups simply bounce back and forth between the phases of pseudo-community and chaos. If you really want to reap significant benefits, you should seek the company of trusted people willing to operate out of emptiness and community.

I'm not against support groups. However, I only support those groups that truly support those with chronic illness and/or their loved ones. Every individual and couple needs to shop around for the right group, just as they would the right doctor. And don't be afraid to try to influence a group so that it provides more of what you need. People who deal directly or indirectly with chronic illness are often low on time and energy. So why waste these limited resources on the easy answer of a support group if it truly is not providing solutions, good fellowship and hope?

Ease Into Chaos

— *or* —

Check Your Motive

Imagine that you love Disneyland, but hate the desert. Let's say you are driving your car from the American Midlands to Anaheim, Calif. You dread the thought of motoring through those endless hours of desert terrain in Utah and Nevada, but realize that this tough stretch is a prerequisite to reaching your Disneyland destination. In the prologue to this book, I gave a brief description of all four phases, including chaos. Phase two includes attributes such as intense conflict, screaming, passive-aggressive put-downs, win/lose struggles, back biting, dishonesty and ineffectiveness. Relatively few people enjoy such an environment. Yet researchers contend that a group must travel through chaos to get to the fourth phase of community.

A key message of this book (and one that parallels the progression from phase one to phase four) is the need to be more open and honest. Remember, I believe that in most cases the histrionics of chaos are preferable to the masquerade of pseudo-community. The insidiously nice phase one is more damaging, in my mind, than the black-cloaked phase two.

Yet, I abhor the rip-snorting chaos that verges on the edge or crosses over the line to verbal, emotional or physical abuse. I urge individuals, couples and groups to escape the pseudo-community phase and enter the realm of chaos while maintaining self-control and respect for others.

The key to a more healthy chaos is to keep motive in mind. In other words, what is your motive or rationale for bringing up what might be a difficult or controversial topic? Let's say that you meet your ill significant other for lunch every Friday at a neighborhood restaurant. You always get there on time. However, like clockwork, your significant other strolls in a few minutes late. You feel tempted to take off the mask and attack the person with brutal honesty. But before you do so, check your motive for wanting to berate your ill partner.

Scenario 1: Perhaps you think about the tardiness and realize that the 10 minutes you are there by yourself provides a pleasant interlude in your day. It gives you a chance to relax by yourself for a few minutes, maybe doing some mental processing of what happened at work, or mentally rehearsing something you want to tell your lunch date. You also realize the person's tardiness has never caused you to be late for work on Friday afternoons. By thinking it over, you realize the person's tardiness is not a big deal. But what if you still want to chastise the person as soon as he or she sits down? "Your tardiness is highly unprofessional and feels like a slap in the face to me!" you might say. At that point your motive is in question. You already determined the tardiness is insignificant. Most likely, you are using the tardiness for an excuse to put the person on the spot for another, unnamed reason. Most people at this point will get defensive and the conversation will spiral quickly into a win-lose struggle.

Scenario 2: You analyze your date's tardiness and come to the conclusion that it is a problem. Perhaps a wave of customers comes right at noon and you and your date must wait several minutes before being seated. Maybe you have missed part of staff meetings at work because you get out of the restaurant late. Maybe your concern about being late to work influences your mood throughout each date, making them less enjoyable than they could be. At this point, you probably have the right motive for bringing up the topic of your date's perpetual lateness. The key now, however, is to approach the subject in a way that breaks out of the comfort of pseudo-community without verbally "beating up on" the other person. How you start that conversation greatly impacts how the entire discussion goes. Here is one way it could begin:

You: Hey, you're late again. This has to stop. You and your tardiness could get me in deep trouble at work.

Yes, your mask is cracking but you have put your lunch date on the defensive. It's easy to imagine his or her response taking the conversation into a more personal, hurtful realm. Sprinkling your conversation with the word "you" – especially if said in an accusatory tone – is a great way to create a me-you, win-lose battle.

Here is another way you could begin the discussion.

You: This is tough for me to say, but I'm a bit confused and angry that our lunch dates start late each week. I know it makes me somewhat uptight because I worry about getting back to work on time. I would like to find out if there is a way we could get started a little earlier so I don't have to worry about making it back to work on time. What are your thoughts?

That kind of lead-in creates an opening for adult-to-adult discussion, real problem solving. Notice that the second lead-in is sprinkled with the pronouns "I" rather than "you." I do

not believe the second lead-in is cowardly or politically correct or phony. I believe it is courageous in that it brings up an
important topic rather than keeping a lid on it. True, there is
likely to be some discomfort caused by the discussion, but
that's a sign you and your date have moved out of the stagnation of the pseudo-community phase. This lead-in sets the
stage for a more effective dialogue.

In the spring of 1995, Sherrie invited me to have lunch
with her at a local restaurant. We sat munching deli sandwiches outside on the establishment's sun-drenched patio.
There had been unspoken tension between us for about a
month. I sensed Sherrie intended to bring the topic to light
during our date, but I would have preferred to avoid any conflict on that gorgeous day. However, in kind, loving and true
words, she told me she missed me, an odd statement considering I had not been on the road during that month. She said
I seemed preoccupied with my business, even when surrounded by family members at the dinner table. She reminded me that there are several different brands of workaholism
and that I seemed in danger of falling into that addictive trap.
But, she also reiterated her love and concern for me.

The conversation made me uncomfortable – a sure sign of
breaking out of phase one. I felt a twinge of anger, but her
words never forced me to get defensive. I mainly listened during that lunch and thought about her words the rest of the
afternoon. I realized she had given five key messages.

1. I love you.
2. I miss you.
3. The kids miss you and need you.
4. I believe you are at risk of becoming a workaholic.

5. Please consider my words and do what's right for you and the family.

Sherrie did not lambaste me. She even brought up the topic in a pleasant environment. She focused on her feelings and her concern for my well being. And she let me decide how to handle the situation. A day later I came up with a plan of action in response to Sherrie's messages and it made me feel as if I had just been released from a minimum-security prison. Thanks to Sherrie's hedging, the first thing I do when I arrive home from work is go to my desk and set my briefcase down on the floor. Then I walk out of the room. I close up shop when I complete that simple ritual. As I walk out of my office I mentally flip off the switch that monitors the professional consultant within me. I can then focus on my personal life the rest of the day.

Sherrie chose to bring an important topic to light that day we met for lunch because she had a good and true motive for discussing it with me. She delivered her message with love and respect, helping us begin to solve one of our many problems. Yes, Sherrie's body is ill but the rest of her is extremely healthy.

Difficult Lessons

— *or* —

"The Fat Lady of Revelation"

Writing a book gives many people a false sense of self-importance. While working on this book at the corner table of a local restaurant I frequent, I acted like a self-important ass to two women sitting at the adjacent table. Restaurants often stimulate my creativity as a writer. The noise and movement of a bustling eatery, combined with my fingers tapping on a notebook computer, make for a wonderful afternoon of work. A crab enchilada and a frosty glass of beer are pleasant additions to this off-site work environment.

However, one of the women at the next table drove me to distraction with her inane and judgmental banter about her co-workers, rotund mothers-in-law, frumpy homemakers and alcoholic relatives. Even the way she sat, with her thin, long foot dangling in the aisle, annoyed me. She apparently had read the latest guide to being a cool professional of the '90s and wanted to make sure everyone within earshot knew it.

I tried covering my ears and closing my eyes to get my thoughts together. Eventually, though, I had to put my fingers on the keyboard as I struggled for creative control against her silky, know-it-all voice that droned against my ears.

Normally I'm a calm guy, but this particular day I needed to let off some steam. In the middle of a diatribe about a friend's mother, she said, "Well I shouldn't say this but . . ."

"Then please don't," I interrupted. "I'm sorry for saying this, but I'm getting irritated having to listen to you go on and on about people who can't defend themselves."

The shocking thing about the woman's reaction was that she did not seem shocked about my reaction to her.

"I just can't get my work done listening in on your galling conversation."

"OK," the woman said, "we'll talk more softly."

I focused on the computer screen, but felt guilty for judging the woman I labeled judgmental. Five minutes after I confronted the woman and her friend, they stood to leave. I said: "I sometimes find it is therapeutic being a jerk, but I don't think it is especially therapeutic for those I treat like a jerk. I apologize."

"Thanks for the apology," said the woman who was the prime target of my rudeness. Her sidekick smiled and nodded. Then they left, leaving me alone with my work and guilt.

The restaurant vignette reminds me of an Alan Jones book titled, *Soul Making: The Desert Way of Spirituality*. Jones refers to angels of God, who often come in the guise of what he calls "The Fat Lady." The author tells the story of Alexander Schmemann, a distinguished Orthodox priest and teacher, who learned an important truth about himself while traveling on a crowded train in Paris. As a young man, Schmemann and his fiancée crammed into a crowded metro. A large, unattractive woman wearing a Salvation Army uniform came aboard and sat next to them. The young couple whispered in Russian to each other about how ugly the woman was. Then the train came to a stop and the large woman arose, saying in perfect

Russian, "I wasn't always ugly!" Schmemann considered her an angel of God because she "brought the shock of revelation, the shock that was needed for me to see that what was there was much, much more than an ugly old woman."

We often cruise down the tracks of life in a funk, failing to observe the landscape around us, staying stuck in the predictability of our routines and beliefs. The woman on the metro forced Schmemann and his fiancée to explore beneath the skin of the stranger and into the depths of their hearts.

I believe "The Fat Lady of Revelation" comes in many shapes and forms. Perhaps I was "The Fat Lady" for the young woman at the restaurant, bringing to her a "shocking revelation" of how others respond to her gossip. I'm sure she disliked my actions and me, but there is a chance she will do a self-assessment regarding the way she belittles others through her words.

Perhaps the petite, professional woman returned the favor by also being my "Fat Lady." She forced me to look at my actions, which were those of an ass. My childhood buddies and I used to say, "A skunk smells its own scent." My judgmental thoughts about the woman whom I considered judgmental spilled over into some cutting spoken words that revealed my own judgmental traits and forced me to consider what I do about them.

"The Fat Lady of Revelation" doesn't always come to us in human form. Sometimes, she is something as egregious and all-encompassing as chronic illness. The "Fat Lady" of chronic illness has at times grabbed Sherrie from behind and forced her to the mat. She has often extinguished all the joy and comfort out of Sherrie's life. In so doing, she has indirectly swatted me upside the head. But this "Fat Lady" of chronic illness has given me a deep, rich picture of Sherrie, life and myself that I had never seen before she entered the scene.

In her book titled *Co-dependent No More*, Melody Beattie wrote: "Everything from our pasts has prepared and propelled us for tomorrow. And it all works out for the good. Nothing's wasted."

The lessons learned from "The Fat Lady" of chronic illness have been hard and cruel. If we fail to learn those lessons, however, our lack of enlightenment can lead our relationships down a dark and sinister path that may lead to trouble and waste.

The woman on the metro said, "I wasn't always ugly." Sherrie has often felt like telling people, "I wasn't always sick." She could also add, "I wasn't always as wise, tender, tough and loving as I am now." I am a slow study, but over the years "The Fat Lady" of chronic illness taught me some tough but valuable lessons about rescue, forgiveness and healing, perseverance and honesty, courage and sacrifice, health and real love. The shocking revelation of chronic illness has propelled me to acquire greater wisdom and strength than ever before.

The "Fat Lady" of chronic illness stirs up a witch's brew of poor health and bitter emotions that challenge the best of relationships. She doesn't spoon feed her students, nor does she force them to put new insight into practice. But when you have such an instructor, you can't help seeing life from a different perspective. You don't have to love or admire "The Fat Lady," but you definitely can learn from her. Benjamin Franklin could have been talking about her when he said, "Those things that hurt, instruct." You must choose whether her presence in your life crushes or strengthens you.

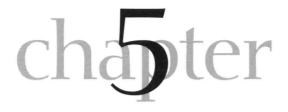

chapter 5

THE "BIG 5" IN PHASE TWO

Notice the stark difference in how people handle these big topics in phase two, as opposed to phase one.

Support:

The Universe is Heliocentric

— or —

Dash the Doubts & the Doubters

For centuries, much of the civilized world knew one thing for sure: The sun and planets circled the earth, which stood firmly at the center of the universe. Then Polish astronomer Nicolaus Copernicus (1473-1543) messed with the minds of mankind, claiming the universe was heliocentric (sun-centered). For those who took the topic seriously, Copernicus might just as naturally have turned their minds and bodies inside out. In a way, he told them black is white, up is down, and forward is backward.

In 1543 Copernicus published a book titled *On the Revolutions of the Heavenly Spheres*, which used scientific observations to justify a heliocentric view. Many of his peers and religious leaders pooh-poohed his work. It took several more decades before a heliocentric philosophy took hold of the scientific community and later the general populace. People don't blithely change their views. Neither do scientific findings or medical diagnoses guarantee a person will change a strongly held view. Many folks clung to an outdated theory about Sherrie's health. She had always been healthy and was far too young to have serious, ongoing problems.

"How's Sherrie?" an acquaintance would ask.

"She's still sick."

"After all these months? Really? Has she tried vitamins?"

People tend to cluster around those who are similar to themselves. We worked and socialized with baby boomers whose idea of chronic illness was a 48-hour flu.

"Can your family come over tonight for dinner?"

"Not tonight. Sherrie has the flu again. Some other time we would love to."

"This is the third time you've said you can't make it."

"Well, I'm sorry. All I can say is she's not doing well tonight so we'd like to take a rain check."

"OK, I'll call in a few days."

The next invitation came four years later.

An extended family member asked for an update on Sherrie's health. She apparently did not comprehend my answer. "Oh, Gregg, do you think it's something else that's bothering her?"

"Like what?"

"I don't know. Uh, are you guys doing OK in your relationship?"

Medical amateurs weren't the only ones who asked that question. At least two doctors, who depended on easy answers, questioned whether Sherrie's illness was psychosomatic. "Have you considered marriage counseling?" one asked. The young, healthy Sherrie would have quipped, "Marriage counseling for a herniated disk?" – which doctors later verified as the cause of the headaches and body pain. The exhausted and sick Sherrie didn't respond till she got home. Then she exploded.

She told one doctor several times that if she exercised more than a minimal amount she felt horrid the next week.

Invariably, his suggestion at the end of each appointment would be to get out of the house more. "Oh," he added, "and be sure to do some regular aerobic exercise."

A classic "Candid Camera" segment showed a person waiting for an elevator. When the door opened, the person saw "Candid Camera" actors facing the back of the elevator. Hesitantly, the person stepped in and, sure enough, faced the rear of the elevator. After a few seconds, the actors turned in unison to the left. The victim of this charade quickly followed suit. Other victims responded the same way. The "victims" of this prank knew to face the front of the elevator. But the herd mentality coaxed them to do something they instinctively knew was wrong.

Sherrie got sick in our 12th year of marriage. We knew much about each other by then. I had lived with her day after day before and after chronic illness intruded in our lives. Ninety-nine percent of the time I believed everything she said about her symptoms. But there were enough doubters that my faith in Sherrie's honesty wavered occasionally.

Sometimes, I would get up on a Saturday morning and see a messy house. As I pushed the vacuum back and forth, my thoughts about the degree of Sherrie's illness vacillated back and forth. At times, I truly wondered if she felt as lousy as she claimed. I wondered if she should be cleaning the floors instead of me. She often said that dealing with her medical problems was her full-time job. Small, evil thoughts flicked through my mind, wishing her job brought money in rather than siphoning it out.

A group or couple moving into the chaos of phase two don't always do so with a violent, dramatic argument. The chaos might occur behind closed doors, with the forming of coalitions, with group members verbally back-stabbing each other. The gray storm clouds of doubt within my mind were a quiet, crafty form of chaos.

Those seeds of doubt crept into my actions toward Sherrie. Once when I was pushing the vacuum back and forth a bit too firmly Sherrie noticed and asked: "Is something wrong, Gregg?"

"No, I'm just trying to get this done quickly so I can relax a bit this weekend," I answered making a sarcastic comment aimed at Sherrie that was also dishonest in its disguise. Yes, something was wrong. I felt beat from the stress of work and family, and the last thing I wanted to do on a Saturday morning was housework.

Sometimes Sherrie would awaken a few minutes later than usual. "I have another migraine," she would say. "Sorry about that," I would say hurriedly. "I have Bret partially ready for school but you're going to have to do the rest. I'm running late for work." My response to her, communicated through different words and a tone of sourness in my voice, was: "Migraine shmygraine, get over it. You've got a little job to do with Bret and I have a big job to do for a Fortune 100 company."

So, how can you deal with doubt in a more effective way? Here are three suggestions.

1. Become heliocentric (sun-centered).

Copernicus, and astronomers such as Galileo, proved the solar system is heliocentric. Yet, even in the face of facts, many people still fluctuated between a sun- and earth-centered belief. Look at the medical facts and your own observations to come to the firm conclusion that your significant other is indeed sick. Others may still doubt the veracity of that sickness, but they are akin to the people who clung to old concepts about the universe. Get over the shock of the illness and continue your journey. This does not mean you have to cave in to the illness and assume your loved one will always be sick. Fight against the illness while still believing it exists. The earth circles the sun and right now your loved one is chronically ill.

2. Become a PR manager.

Every major company or big-time politician hires an astute public relations manager to help convey key messages to the public. You can play such a role for your significant other. Speaking as a former corporate PR manager, it is important to have a key fact that flavors messages you give doubters. My key fact became: "Yes, Sherrie is definitely sick, but she's one courageous woman who is moving ahead." Remember, this statement is something I try to recall when "doubters" talk to me. I am NOT saying to keep in mind always that your significant other is sick. That leads to sticking the label "patient" on your loved one and all the problems that label brings with it.

Doubter: "I just wonder if it's something more mental that is keeping her from getting well?"

Me/PR Manager: "Sherrie is the wisest and bravest person I know. More than anyone in the world, she wants to get well. Doctors have diagnosed her problems and, unfortunately, some people never fully recover from her type of illness."

Not only do answers such as this support your loved one, they also keep the seeds of doubt from being transplanted from others' heads into yours.

3. Become more truthful.

This tip becomes easier to follow if you also abide by the first two tips. I'm not angry while pushing the vacuum because

I question whether Sherrie is truly sick. I'm angry because I feel dog tired.

"Is something wrong, Gregg?"

I switch off the vacuum. "Yeah, I feel tired. I guess I didn't want to start the weekend like this."

"Well, I can live with a messy house this weekend if you can. Maybe we should do something fun as a couple or as a family."

"That sounds good, but how and when do we get the house cleaned up?"

"How about asking the kids to take care of their rooms and you and I can tackle the rest of the house sometime this weekend. We'll do it just before or just after we do something fun. I'll bet we'll feel better doing it later today."

In this scenario, I did not directly or indirectly attack Sherrie. I gave her a chance to use her creativity to solve a problem. I also got a reprieve from doing the cleaning first thing on a Saturday morning and together we made plans to do something fun.

In summary, perhaps the worst thing I can do for Sherrie is doubt her. She can handle my anger or sadness about her illness because we now operate more out of phases three and four rather than phases one and two. My doubt, however, could be just as debilitating to her as any of her symptoms. My visible and ongoing belief in her is a crucial part of her healing process. Silence your doubts and the doubters.

Medical Maze:
A New Kind of "Caretaker"

— or —

The Dragon Slayer

While slaves were building one of the pyramids, one of them wrote on a wall, "No one was angry enough to speak out."

My early childhood adventures occurred totally in my mind. My brother, cousins and I rode stallions and wore capes as we rescued kindergarten damsels in distress. Every night I drifted to sleep in the midst of another dangerous and courageous adventure. However, in the past 13 years since Sherrie became ill, my life has been more like "Meet the Press" than "Zorro" on the excitement meter. I also learned early on that a worthy life goal is to have everyone like me. That goal is a perfect match for someone trying to fulfill the job description of a "caretaker." Remember, "caretakers" are to be stoical, noncomplaining and polite as they go about their business of being do-gooders. An image of a pressure cooker with all the holes plugged comes to mind. If that baby is on with the holes plugged, you'll eventually get chili blasted all over the wall.

Most Americans grew up learning that doctors are god-like. You don't argue with gods, especially those higher beings who can shorten or prolong your life. When doctors speak, you listen. No back talking. No inane questions. Shut up, listen, and do what they say. Sherrie was sick year after year and saw a line-up of medical specialists for a variety of physical problems. She struggled with pain and exhaustion and felt confused part of the time because of her symptoms and the drugs prescribed. She needed help from someone as she interacted with the doctor deities. That someone was me – the man who wanted others to like him, the stoical partner who fit the job description of "caretaker" perfectly. And I played the meek "caretaker" role well, nodding my head as doctors spoke, thanking them profusely for their expertise and concern. I even chuckled when they practiced examination-room humor.

But one day, when we went to visit another specialist to try to determine the cause of Sherrie's physical problems, I decided to trash that "worthy goal" of being liked. I decided to uncover the pressure-cooker holes. As the specialist asked the same questions other doctors had asked, Sherrie retold the story for what seemed the hundredth time. He probed her mind with questions and her body with fingers. He seemed as tired of Sherrie's story and problems as we were. He answered our questions with curt statements, refusing to look us in the eyes. Then he said it was time for us to go. I was still learning how to allow others to dislike me, so I simply did as directed. He told us he would call in a day or two with his diagnosis.

So I took my wife of 14 years home. I watched her walk stiffly from room to room. I saw her blank face stare into the eyes of our beloved daughters. I watched her wince in pain as she reached down to pick up our tiny old dog who seemed as tired as she did. I wondered why the wife of my youth had vanished.

Two days later Sherrie received a call from the doctor. When I walked in the door from work Sherrie was storming around the house like a professional wrestler, although she still felt as if chronic illness had her in a full-nelson grip. "The doctor wondered how things are going between you and me," she said angrily. "He suggested we see a marriage counselor. He thought I needed to get out of the house more and that I might consider signing up for some exercise classes." Then she retold the doctor's coup d'etat. "He doesn't think I have anything physically wrong with me at all. He just thinks I'm a little bit depressed." She spoke her last words as if she were telling me that a con man had swindled her out of her last nickel.

The old Gregg Piburn – the one everyone liked, the one who considered doctors gods, the one who fit the "caretaker" bill perfectly, the one who resided in the pseudo-community phase – would have said: "Now now, Sherrie. I think he made a mistake but there's no use getting upset about it. We'll make an appointment to see another doctor tomorrow. Let's go watch TV." Good little Greggie. The perfect and polite "caretaker."

This time I chose a different route and let steam spew from the pressure cooker I had become. Without saying a word, I marched to the phone. "Yes," I said into the phone, "let me talk to the doctor." Pause. "This is very important so I need to talk to him now."

I waited for two minutes while the person at the other end of the line tracked down the doctor. Finally, he came on the line. I asked him to quickly summarize what he had told Sherrie. Her recollection matched his summary. Then it was my turn to talk.

"I've lived with this woman for 14 years and I guarantee there is something significantly wrong with her body," I said through clenched teeth. Sherrie stood by me, her eyes growing wide. "We are both offended that you would belittle her and her illness by saying what you said." The doctor began to interrupt. "Be quiet, let me speak for once," I countered. "You treated Sherrie with disinterest two days ago and you've upset her with your idiotic diagnosis today. If anyone is sick in the head it's you. If I ever hear you question Sherrie's honesty or toughness again, I'll punch you in the mouth." I slammed down the phone.

I broke all the rules . . . and I loved it. So did Sherrie. My explosion turned what could have been a sour evening into a grand affair as we joked and laughed about the doctor and the tongue-lashing. Did I really intend to punch out the doctor? Not likely, because I hoped our paths would never cross again. And luckily they haven't.

This may sound crazy, especially if you operate according to the behavior patterns of the pseudo-community phase, but allowing others to dislike me represented personal growth. More important than that, however, my actions supported Sherrie in a new and bizarre way. She did not need a pat on the back at that moment. She did not need a quintessential "caretaker" to bring her warm soup while her mind smoldered with anger and questions about her sanity. She needed a knight in shining armor to stand up for her, a princely figure willing to look square into the eyes of the dragon dressed in a doctor's smock. She needed someone to be angry and speak out. She needed someone to slay the dragon.

Parenting:
Chaos as Catalyst

— or —

A Hole in the Wall

Sherrie and I were in the kitchen preparing breakfast when Corlet walked in, still wearing pajamas. "Before you eat," Sherrie said, matter-of-factly, "please put your dirty dishes from last night into the dishwasher."

"I don't have time," she responded in a sassy voice. "I have to get ready for school."

"Come on, help your mom out," I said.

"No," she said with finality as she walked between the counter and a microwave oven. As she passed, I put my hand around her upper arm – not hard, but firm enough to keep her from walking away from us.

"Wait a minute," I said in a slow, baritone voice. But before I finished my statement to insist she put the dirty dishes away and apologize to Sherrie, she jerked her arm out of my grasp. Her triceps brushed against the oven handle and she started screaming as if I had belted her with a boxer's right cross.

"That is child abuse," she yelled and started to storm out of the kitchen.

"No an accidental scratch is NOT child abuse!" I yelled as I reached for her other arm and firmly, but nonviolently, coaxed her onto a chair in the dining room. I stooped down within a few inches of my 12-year-old daughter's eyes and saw primal fear emanating from her face. This vision of Corlet's angelic face contorted with fright broke my heart. It was evident that Corlet's behavior was something more than a typical pubescent outburst. Sherrie's chronic conditions, along with the other vagaries of life in the '90s, had frayed the nerves of everyone in the family. During a second or two of silence, I felt as if the earth had rolled to the edge of a dark precipice, teetering on a dime. I held my breath, wondering if the earth would roll back to safety or edge ahead and fall into the infernal black hole and I watched Corlet's face change from fear to disgust.

"Don't . . . ever . . . touch . . . me . . . again," she hissed.

Then I felt the earth slip over the edge. My glasses flew off my face as I jerked backward at the waist. I screamed the primitive scream of a Neanderthal Man looking to the heavens while feeling like hell. I thought, "This is what I get for busting my butt to provide love and support to my family?!"

The Neanderthal within screamed one more time as I backhanded the dining-room wall, leaving a dent the size of a paperback book. Corlet's face had turned from disgust to shock and Sherrie stood looking at me with a strong dose of resignation mixed with a pinch of relief. Then I saw 10-year-old Alyse running up the stairs with fear in her eyes and tears on her cheeks. That was the image – the countenance of my beloved and innocent daughter – that turned my spirit from anger to sorrow.

I slumped into a nearby chair, put my elbows onto my knees and sobbed into my hands. The sound of a grown man sobbing is as foreign to most families as hearing a coyote howl in the kitchen. My wife and daughters froze as this strange sound permeated the room. Then Sherrie came and knelt in front of me, putting her arms around my neck and whispering, "It's OK, it's OK, it's OK, it's OK." Her simple and loving words fueled a few more seconds of sobs before the crying died out.

I looked up with red eyes and noticed my girls still sat and stood where they had been but they no longer showed signs of fear. "Come here, girls," Sherrie said, "we need to talk." They came slowly, like stray dogs unsure about a kind hand holding food scraps. Then the three females I love the most sat on the floor in front of me, while I explained why I exploded. I told them how difficult life seemed to be for everyone in the family lately. I confessed my hatred for child abusers. But mostly, I told them how sad I felt about Sherrie's ongoing medical problems. Group hugs in a business setting can be phony. The group hug the four of us did that morning was the real thing.

To get from phase one to phase four, you have to go through phases two and three. For those comfortably familiar with the equilibrium of the pseudo-community phase, the chaos and conflict my family and I experienced that fateful morning seems foreign and obscene. However, without the rage of chaos we would not have ventured into the vulnerable phase of emptiness. The morning took on a life of its own, one that included honesty, emotion, vulnerability and closeness. All four of us learned something important about one another that would not have occurred had we stayed in our safe cocoon of pseudo-community.

The scene included no physical abuse. Some might question whether anyone was emotionally abused. If I had slammed the wall and immediately walked out of the house, then I might be guilty. Instead, we acknowledged through our words and actions that life is difficult and we will walk the rocky path together, in love. I chose to keep the dent in the wall for several months. We used it as a symbol of the pain, and the love, we shared then and to this day.

Intimacy:

Cold as Ice

— *or* —

Hot Tips

L isten up, class. Today we begin our sex-education unit of the course. Hey, stop that! There will be no giggling in my class. Now, pay attention, especially if you happen to be someone who is a lover of a person who is chronically ill.

Fact #1: Certain people are frigid in bed.

This is not an in-depth study of this phenomenon. Let us just say that some people do not care for sexual intimacy or have a hard time responding with interest and energy to the act of lovemaking.

Fact #2: Feeling rotten causes temporary sexual frigidity in virtually all people.

I'm not talking about having the sniffles preventing you from making love. I'm talking about laid-low-flat-out-sick-get-food-out-of-my-sight-I-think-I-want-to-die-my-eyeballs-are-about-to-burst-did-anyone-get-the-license-plate-number-of-that-Mack-truck sick. This should come as no surprise. After all, when significantly ill (even if only for a day or two) you don't want to do things such as attend a Broadway play, hike a beautiful mountain trail or make love to your lover. Your body is out of commission as it seeks rest and recovery.

Fact #3: Healthy bed partners often feel frisky and are in for a big disappointment.

Don't get the idea I was constantly pawing Sherrie during her bouts with various maladies. Through most stages of her illness, she has been willing and able to have sex, although not as regularly as when she was healthy. There were times, such as after Sherrie underwent spine surgeries, when we refrained from sex for weeks at a time. The bad news and good news is that during all of these "down" times, I still felt sexually attracted to my wife. So when I got my hopes up and then found out she could not have sex, I felt frustrated and sometimes angry.

Fact #4: There are bad and good ways to respond to that anger and frustration.

Let's take a brief look at a few of those negative and positive ways.

Option #1: You could go elsewhere for satisfaction.

This gets down to the nitty-gritty of morality. I consider this option wrong. It also adds more stress to an already shaky relationship rocked by chronic illness. If married, it also contradicts vows you likely made at a wedding ceremony. Call me old-fashioned, but vows demand more commitment than idle banter. "Hey, let's commit to a faithful relationship for as long as we both live." "Sounds great, let's give it a shot." A true vow is much more sincere and powerful than "let's give it a shot."

Option #2: You could seek different kinds of physical satisfaction with your lover.

Sherrie needed to know I found her attractive even when she felt awful. I could say it but I also needed (and wanted!) to show that her body attracted me. Warm, unexpected hugs and long, gentle kisses brought us intimacy without having to go the distance. Sometimes I would tell Sherrie from the start that I knew we would not be able to "do it," but still needed to be close to her. This allowed her to relax and enjoy our short sexual encounters. Sometimes that relaxation and enjoyment would lead to a change in plans and we would end up going the distance. But I let Sherrie lead the way and she knew she could back off at any time.

Option #3: You could physically force yourself on your lover.

This is rape, which can occur in a marriage as well as between strangers. You can plead and cajole before finally forcing the person to have sex with you. This is chaos of the worst type. It portrays the sensitivity of a beast, hardly the kind of support needed by a loved one who is chronically ill.

Option #4: You could go all the way in a different way.

Warm hugs and gentle kisses feel good at the time, but might only lead down a dead-end alley. For a man, the arousal might necessitate ejaculation. Without it, the night seems wasted. These may be harsh words, but it could be reality in many cases. Masturbation seems a fine alternative to me. Some people feel guilty about this. But I suggest that you talk openly to your lover about it. I believe you'll develop some creative solutions that take the pressure off your ill lover and provide you with a satisfying physical release.

Option #5: You could mentally neuter yourself.

Men and women are spiritual, mental and physical beings. Part of the "caretaker" mentality is to deny your feelings and pleasures while protecting your little "china doll." By denying yourself sexual intimacy, you are also denying sexual pleasures for your lover. You make him or her feel unattractive and unwanted. The Option 5 approach assumes an all-or-nothing philosophy about sex. There are many wonderful and loving pleasures between those two extremes on the continuum.

Option #6: You could mentally open yourself up to richer, creative pleasures.

Some of you reading this book earn livings solving problems creatively. Chronic illness often creates sexual problems in a partnership and can be solved quite easily if people put their creativity to work in the bedroom. Sherrie and I found our creative solutions often were simple ones. As we chose to learn and grow from her illness, we found our love for each other became stronger. A simple squeeze of the hand while walking in the mall or an unhurried foot rub after a long day took on new meaning in our adapted lives. As I became more gentle and attuned to Sherrie's body and needs, the greater became our love for one another, which resulted in more fulfilling lovemaking.

The odd-numbered options above portray people operating out of chaos and/or pseudo-community. The even-numbered options describe ways to handle a difficult situation above the barbed wire – in the emptiness and community phases. Chronic illness might limit your sexual activities. However, the approach you and a lover take to those limitations might have just as significant an impact on your sex life as the illness itself. Open up the lines of communication about sex and see what vistas await you and your lover on the other side of the barbed wire.

Spiritual:
Be Real to Find Real

– or –

Mad at God

Does God exist? I hate to disappoint you, but you won't find the definitive answer to that question in the pages of this book. Determining whether God is real is a personal quest depending much more on faith than facts.

Unfortunately, God is not real in the sense that you can kiss him, hug him, pinch him or slap him. So determining his existence must deal in the realm of intangibles, things you can't see or touch. You flat-out can't see a photograph of him or make an appointment to meet him next Tuesday at his office. You can see aspen leaves shake in the wind, but you can't see the wind that creates the movement. Likewise, you can see the aspen tree, but not God or some other force that created the seed that grew into that tree. You can't force God to come out of hiding, even if he is real. You can see two friends throwing a football back and forth at the park. The activity gives evidence of a relationship between two people. But you can't see the relationship, only the expressions and results of it. Many unseen forces – wind, relationships, hope, electricity, love, speed, fear and, perhaps, God, if he exists – affect our lives daily. But in various ways, we have to play a participatory role for each to be real in our lives. We have to open our heart to a lover, turn on the light switch and move our bodies in the act of lovemaking.

I sometimes help corporate executives prepare for and deliver effective presentations. As part of their preparation, I ask them to consider this question: "After the presentation, how do you want your audience members to feel?" One executive might respond, "anxious." Another might say, "hopeful." A third might answer, "excited." I tell them that to achieve that goal, they have to emit, through words and actions, the feeling they desire their audience to display. If a presenter fails to show excitement during his presentation, he can't expect his audience to feel that emotion. Similarly, how can God be real if you aren't real?

As I said in the last chapter, relationships are more important than rules in my perception of religion. Strong relationships thrive and survive by people being real, by people doing and saying what's really on their mind. Strong relationships are also created when people are courageous enough to be honest and wise enough to do so without causing irreparable damage to others.

How can God be real if you aren't real?

"Oh Lord, I beseech thee to have mercy on my wife, a gift from you who now labors under the heavy burden of chronic illness. I know thou must have mysterious reasons beyond my feeble comprehension for permitting her body to deteriorate while she is still so young. But you are a great God who makes all things good and right. I trust that Sherrie and I are living within your will, playing out the role you have determined for

our lives. Thank you for allowing us to be performers in your Great Play of Life. Give Sherrie a sense of joy about each day, even when she feels trapped by unseen forces that strip her of energy and prick her with pain. Help me, Lord, to be a godly ambassador of your love and wisdom as I seek to support Sherrie in a most loving way. Thank you for the gift of life and the hope of tomorrow. Amen."

Intellectually I believe some of the statements in the prayer above. I confess that in the early years of Sherrie's sickness I mainly communicated with God in the flowery language demonstrated above. I thought that was how I SHOULD speak to God. I thought that was how I showed God I was a good and spiritual person. I created a nice and polite pseudo-community relationship with God. I ignored my emotions and refrained from being vulnerable. I belittled Sherrie's illness, I belittled Sherrie, I belittled myself and I belittled God. I claimed to adhere to religious beliefs based on a strong relationship, but I refused to be real with God. I had created a mediocre and mundane religion void of energy, power and life.

One night, long after Sherrie and the kids had gone to bed, I started to walk to the desk in the family room. I had set aside 20 minutes nightly to read the Bible and pray. Before I got to the desk, I fell to my knees and put my head on the seat of a recliner chair. I started to sob. These words shot invisibly from my brain to God, wherever he was. "What the hell are you trying to prove, God? How much is Sherrie supposed to withstand? I'm getting sick of her sickness and I'm getting sick of your decision to keep her sick. If this is some stupid heavenly game, I give up. I give up! You win. We lose.

Leave us alone, God. You are not helping one bit. Go ambush some other ignorant couple. I've had it with you."

The stream of words dried up and I sat still, surrounded by a comforting silence. Lightning bolts did not zap me nor did guilty feelings overwhelm me. For the first time in a long while I felt God's presence. He became more real to me because I was real with him. And in the silence following my internal chaos, I sensed he would be with us whatever happened. I sensed he would help Sherrie and me grow in the midst of her illness.

Before I stood up and went to bed, I said softly, "I really need you God."

In a classic scene from the movie "Jerry Maguire," the two protagonists have an argument in a locker room. Jerry Maguire, the sports agent, is trying to persuade Rod Tillman, an Arizona Cardinal wide receiver who is his client, to have a more positive attitude on the field and with fans. The men wander through all four phases as they meander through the locker room. Finally, the conversation becomes too uncomfortable for Jerry and he says, "I'll see you in Phoenix." He walks away. The last image shows Rod, stark naked, holding up his arms and saying with a smile, "You think we're arguing and I think we're just starting to communicate." My first prayers about Sherrie's illness were phony, pointless arrows shot into a void. My latter prayers, pointed and real, hit the mark. I have been the real Gregg communicating with a real God ever since.

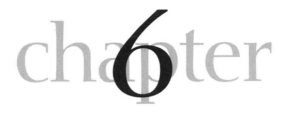

chapter **6**

CHAOS
PRODUCES
CHANGE

Pseudo-community residents fight change
as they seek the comfortable status quo.
Notice how phase two helps create real
change.

A Sickening "Compliment"

— or —

The Chameleon

I sat in my boss's cubicle looking at potted plants on book shelves. The vegetation seemed as misplaced as I felt in that corporate setting. But the Swedish ivy seemed far more alive than I did at that moment. My boss and I chatted about a variety of issues – an upcoming media event, the quality of a GM's recent presentation, the chances of the Broncos having a winning season, the need for me to produce charts proving my work efforts brought value to the organization. Other than the Broncos discussion, I felt strangely disinterested in the rest of the topics. My mind drifted to the edge of the universe, a dark void. Then, as if to awaken me from long slumber, my boss slipped a phrase into the conversation that left me puzzled.

"Well, everybody likes Gregg Piburn," he said. He didn't mean it literally, although there was a good dose of truth to the statement. "Well," I said with a silly Gomer Pyle grin, "I don't know about that." He changed the subject again and we talked for another five minutes about another mundane topic, but nothing else he said to me got through. His "compliment" stuck to my brain like flypaper. As I took the 60-second walk back to my cubicle, I felt as if a 100-pound helmet inscribed with the word "Paradox" was perched on my head.

I knew everyone did not like me, but I also knew I wanted everyone I met to do so. I knew that having everyone like me had been an unwritten goal of mine since I was a snot-nosed toddler clinging to Mom. Yet, I knew that my boss's words – which should have been validation of a life lived well, according to my lifelong philosophy – gave me a strange sensation, as if receiving a promotion to a job I was not sure I wanted.

I had an hour to kill before completing my eight-hour work detainment, so I sat with my feet propped up on the desk in my cubicle dissecting my boss's words in my mind as if they were a frog in 10th-grade biology. And when I peeled back all the layers of meaning my boss's words carried, I made a strange finding. I did not see a dead frog but a live chameleon – me. If virtually everyone likes me, I whispered to myself, then who the hell am I? An answer popped into my head: I was a two-legged, upright chameleon. Just as a chameleon changes color to increase its odds of survival, I said and did things to improve the odds of others liking me. My transformation involved popularity and comfort, rather than life and death. I found it more comfortable for others, and myself, if I simply fit in. And I believed others liked me more when I followed their script.

Driving home that afternoon, still mulling over my boss's words in my mind, I thought about whether I had a philosophy of parenting. Before I drove into the driveway at the end of my commute, I realized I did have a philosophy, but I had never put it into words. "I want my kids to like me now and forever," I said silently to myself. "I want them to become old people who will look back on their 'Cool Dad.' I looked back at some of my behavior of the past, some of those times when

I chose the easy route of parenting rather than taking a tough stand. I saw myself wearing a placard that said, 'Hey, kids, please like me!'"

I felt like puking. No wonder I played the role of "caretaker" so well. I relished the kudos I received from others for being so tireless, so selfless, so supportive of Sherrie and the kids. Who wouldn't like an uncomplaining saint or martyr? Sure, sometimes my kids complained about how I acted so perfect, so in control, but I knew deep down they really liked me. They just needed to blow off some steam, I guessed. (Of course I didn't – I thought. I just needed people to like me.) I needed to fulfill that strong urge to fit the "job description" of "caretaker" like a well-tailored sports coat. I deserved recognition as pseudo-community citizen of the decade.

I realized the falsity of my boss's words. How could everyone like Gregg Piburn, when Gregg Piburn didn't truly exist? He was nothing more than a hall of mirrors, mere reflections of what others wanted him to be. He was a do-gooder phantom who wore interchangeable personalities designed to please everyone but himself. Later that night, while my family slept, I made a vow to begin understanding who I really was and what I really believed. I also developed my first goal for that endeavor. I wanted some people to dislike me. Did you read me loud and clear? I WANTED some people to DISLIKE me. That became my goal rather than an abhorrent situation I hoped to prevent. Put that in your "caretaker" pipe and smoke it.

However, that did not mean I wanted one or more of my children to dislike me for the rest of their lives, for example. What happened is that I became willing to have a child, parent, friend, stranger or Sherrie dislike me at any given moment.

It also did not mean I would now go out and steal purses from kindly spinsters or spit in the faces of incompetent high-school referees. It meant that I chose to let the real Gregg Piburn, the one who had evolved over recent years, have his say without worrying about whether others liked him. I chose to be a "lizard" willing to stay with one color and to be true to that color. "You know," my buddy John said one day on one of our afternoon junkets, "I like you much better when you let me see your darker side, when you don't try to be so perfect."

My family and I moved to a new neighborhood on Dec. 19, 1997. A week after our move, I heard that the neighbor behind us yelled at Bret and a friend for being on some rocks that apparently are on his property rather than ours. A month later, Alyse and two of her friends were cross-country skiing in deep snow around our house. Unknowingly, they got onto this precious rock pile. As I walked into the backyard to bring one of the girls a pair of gloves, I saw our neighbor come onto his porch and scream, "Get off those rocks!"

The new Gregg Piburn dislikes adults treating teenagers as sub-humans. The new Gregg Piburn, who doesn't mind being disliked himself, yelled: "Hey, we moved here two months ago and all I've heard from you is screaming at my kids! Thanks for welcoming us into the neighborhood!" He looked at me dumbfounded, then waved his hand at me as if I were nothing more than an irritating fly. I walked into the house and looked in the mirror. I didn't see a fly or a chameleon staring back at me and I didn't see a "caretaker" or a creep. I saw myself, and the image was more clear than it had ever been.

Clip "The Question"

— or —

How Are YOU Doing?

*H*ow *is Sherrie doing?*

Chaos occurs in many forms. Yes, it can mean screaming at a neighbor, or punching a hole in the dining-room wall, or having Sherrie say she's angry at me for a reason she can't quite pinpoint.

How is Sherrie doing?

Chaos also reveals itself in less dramatic forms. One way to determine if you have moved from the pseudo-community phase to the chaos phase is to check your comfort level. If there's discomfort, you have likely risen to phase two.

How is Sherrie doing?

Chaos sometimes comes as a wolf dressed in sheep's clothing. The intent of another person seems honorable, but the reality of his or her words or actions rubs a nerve the wrong way.

How is Sherrie doing?

The words or actions might truly be noble. But if these kind words and actions merge with those of others, over and over, week after week, they become tiny darts that irritate and sting.

How is Sherrie doing?

Since 1985 a zillion people have asked me that question. I'm sick of hearing "The Question" as I've come to call it and I'm tired of hearing myself blab on and on about Sherrie's latest difficulties. Peoples' incessant queries into my wife's status of well being became a tiny dart thrown at me countless times.

A major message throughout this book is to open up the channels of communication wider than ever before. Talk honestly with friends and loved ones about your thoughts and feelings regarding chronic illness and its ramifications. When speaking with a loved one who is sick, dig deep down into issues related to the health problems. Be willing to bust way out of the pseudo-community phase by talking with your loved one about the challenges and impact of chronic illness. Communication will enrich the relationship and help both individuals handle the situation in a healthier manner.

But when it comes to answering "The Question" posed by acquaintances or strangers, I have a different suggestion. Keep the answer short and simple.

Many people in our community know Sherrie and me directly or indirectly. They know that Sherrie has struggled with fibromyalgia and other health issues for years. Often mere acquaintances or strangers have posed "The Question" to me. In the early days, I responded to such queries in great detail. Listeners would respond in one of two ways.

Response #1: Their eyes would glaze over. I came across like Great Aunt Beulah talking about her bout with bunions.

Response #2: The listener would really get into the topic and ask follow-up questions that led to long and dreary discussions ending with my eyes glazed over instead. As an extra penalty, these listeners would sometimes use the conversation with me as a springboard to call Sherrie to offer unwanted advice or convey their own similar problems. And they would invariably call in the middle of one of Sherrie's naps.

If a person is simply being friendly when asking about Sherrie's health, I give a quick response, such as, "She's doing pretty well and thanks for asking." If possible, I walk away at that point or change the topic. My words and actions convey that I am ending the discussion about Sherrie's health. I know some people have felt somewhat put off by my curt reply. Perhaps I seem rude. I don't care. Dealing with Sherrie's chronic conditions saps enough energy out of me as it is. This strategy minimizes time involved talking about how Sherrie feels, especially when there is little potential for a decent return on that investment of time (I sound like the management consultant that I am, don't I?). In addition, if you spend lots of time talking with strangers and acquaintances about your partner's illness, you and others may end up overemphasizing that invisible label of "patient" that has been placed on your loved one.

The other reason to be careful about saying too much is that it can bring you down on a regular basis. Some days three or four people ask me about Sherrie's health. Detailed answers provide constant reminders of a portion of my life that is definitely challenging. It makes me sad to be reminded of Sherrie's problems so often. Too many reminders don't help Sherrie or me. You might be wondering if I'm being hypocritical. I say to be curt while at the same time writing a book about the topic of chronic illness. The thing to remember is that this book does not answer the question, "How is Sherrie doing?" This book responds to the question, "How am I doing?" It answers the question, "How does someone in a relationship with another person who is chronically ill cope with all the challenges of that ordeal successfully?"

There might be times, however, when you want to share more in-depth thoughts and feelings as a response to "The Question." Choose those times carefully. You have enough going on in your life without having to give frequent and lengthy health updates for various people. Do everyone a favor by keeping your answers concise and conclusive. By the way, here's how you can freak out "caretakers" of those who are ill. Go up to them and ask, "Hey, how are YOU doing?" Once they get over the shock, listen intently.

Screaming Cells

— *or* —

Emotional Siamese Twins

Earlier in the day I razzed my friend Dave who confessed he had slept little the night before his daughter's big basketball game. My daughter played in the same four-team tournament that determined the final league standings. His daughter's team lost in the opening round and I figured he would sleep even less tonight. I felt I was above all of that insane whooping and hollering that so many dads do at their children's games. I consider myself a student (hrumph, hrumph), rather than a rabid fan, of basketball.

Yet, eight hours after putting myself on a pedestal, I found myself lying in the fetal position on my bed four hours before bedtime. True, my daughter's team lost in the title game, but that was not why I felt so depressed. Being a former athlete myself, I knew the outcome of one particular game would likely have little or no effect on my daughter's overall life. Yet, I felt her sorrow, and therein lies a clue to why I became such a hard-core "caretaker."

My daughter is a good middle-school athlete who has the potential to become an excellent high-school and college athlete. She might also choose other avenues for her future that take her away from sports. I can live with that. But what was hard to live with today was seeing her coach forget her in the championship game. You see, making it to the title game seemed a wonderful exclamation point to the season for Alyse. She had been a starter all season long and is an excellent playmaker. Despite the fact she played well in the first half, she sat out all but three minutes of the closely contested second half.

Her team may have lost, but her teammates could feel good about how well they performed throughout the season and in the tourney. But Alyse did not and could not feel good about herself based on what happened in the last, most important, game of the year. Her gloom became my gloom.

A year ago, I took one of those personality tests completed by so many corporate executives. My test results revealed an extremely strong tendency to respond to people and events more on an emotional than intellectual level. I'm positive those results would have been much different, more weighted toward the intellect, had I taken the test before starting the grief process related to Sherrie's chronic illness. More relevant and surprising than the general findings however, was Gail's (the test consultant) interpretation of my test scores.

"Gregg, your emotional Geiger counter is probably too strong," she said. "Now I understand why you seem to have such insight about this particular organization that has hired you as a part-time consultant. You walk into a building and quickly get a sense of the collective mood of a group."

I felt a tinge of pride when I heard her interpretation. I agreed that it helped explain my success as an organizational consultant. Then Gail, who knew about Sherrie's illness, took a stab at how my Geiger counter likely plays itself out at home. "I believe when you come home to a family in distress, every cell of your body feels the emotions within the house," she said. "You don't just analyze the situation and think about it. If your wife or daughters or son is hurting, every cell of your body screams that you hurt also." My eyes and heart winced simultaneously as she said those words.

Certain times of my life seem to vibrate with tension, making me as sensitive to the day's happenings as a military scout leading a battalion through the jungle. The spring of 1997, when Gail talked to me, represented one of those high-strung periods. When I came home at night, after work, and put my hand on the doorknob of our front door, I would hesitate, take a deep breath, and wonder what I would find on the other side of the wooden door. Sometimes I entered to siblings screaming at each other, while other days they would be laughing. Sometimes I found Sherrie happily reading to Bret while other days mother and son would be nose to nose like an infuriated manager of a baseball team and an obstinate umpire. An invisible syringe would inject me with the emotions of family members the first 30 seconds after my arrival.

"Emotional sensitivity – like anything else – can be dangerous if used to the extreme," Gail said. "It must be extremely tough to be influenced so much by everything and everyone around you."

Water is a good thing. Without water we all die. Yet, if I fall out of a boat in the middle of a lake, surrounded by all that good wet stuff, I will die. I'm a sinker, not a floater. To care about others is also a good thing. Without compassion, we discard one of those wondrous characteristics that make us human. But too much compassion – which can result in a person assuming the emotions of those around them – can overwhelm us to the point of inaction. Who knows, over the course of decades it might even kill us prematurely.

More than anything, I wanted Alyse to overcome her gloom, to understand that her coach, another imperfect human being, blew it. He admitted that when I chatted with him after the game. So I spent part of the evening in the fetal position, emotionally paralyzed and physically inert. The cells of my body screamed in anguish, then moaned in defeat.

After everyone had gone to bed that night, I woke up and went to check on Alyse. I peeked in and found her sleeping peacefully and I hoped her disappointment of this afternoon had already vanished, that it was not just resting, too. I realize that tomorrow Alyse needs to know I love her unconditionally. No lectures, just acts of love. That is the same kind of appropriate caring my wife needs all the time – whether her symptoms are active or dormant.

It seems wise and helpful for me to tune in to Sherrie's emotions so that I know better how to react to her at any given moment. What seems foolish and harmful is to take on Sherrie's emotions. When I do that, I sometimes take on some of her symptoms, such as exhaustion and depression. When Sherrie is at her lowest, she doesn't need an emotional Siamese twin. She needs someone who will listen and respect her and someone who might occasionally help her rise above the muck. Helping a loved one who is sick is challenging. Trying to help that person while taking on those same emotions and symptoms is probably impossible. I now focus on validating Sherrie's feelings without striving to duplicate them. That's a case of being sensitive *and* smart.

"Caretaker" for Rent

— *or* —

The Affair Affair

If you are a decent plumber for the Acme Plumbing Co., you can likely be an adequate plumber for XYZ Plumbing Co., too. Charles Barkley can dominate a basketball game whether he is in the uniform of the Philadelphia 76ers, the Phoenix Suns or the Houston Rockets. And a person who plays the role of "caretaker" well – as defined by society – can do his or her duties for more than one person. The first two examples are relatively benign, the last example can spell danger for two lovers.

The myth goes like this. Two strangers spot one another across a crowded room. Their eyes lock, at the same moment their hearts intertwine. The physical attraction between the strangers is so strong that romantic feelings carry them to bed within hours, just as surely as the Mississippi River flows into the Gulf of Mexico. This is how affairs begin, so goes the myth.

Sara, as I'll call her, called a week ago and left me a voice mail message. I finally called her this afternoon. She's not doing well. When I met her six years ago, she was a healthy and confident woman who worked with me on a community project. Rheumatoid arthritis now toys with her like a farm cat plays with a field mouse.

The myth is wrong. Most affairs occur between friends rather than strangers. Replace the crowded room with a corporate office or the neighborhood library or the church fellowship hall. A man and a woman strike up a friendship. Yes, there might be a physical attraction at the first meeting, but it causes no concern since it's just two adults getting acquainted. One or both of them are married. But, hey, what's wrong with a little conversation between two consenting adults? The next time they meet, they strike up the conversation right where they left off. Now, when they head to the office or the library or the church, they can't help thinking about each other.

I was one of the first people Sara told about her disease. She sensed I would be sensitive to her plight because I had told her about Sherrie's condition early on in our friendship. After all, to convey the essence of who I was to a new friend, I had to talk about Gregg "the caretaker" and Sherrie "the patient."

"Hey," one of the new friends says, "we ought to get together for lunch sometime." Why limit this new friendship to seemingly chance meetings at one location. "Sure, that would be great." They get together and discover they have even more in common than they had imagined. Both of them leave this first "date" with a new thought: I can really talk with my new friend.

Sara is shy and petite. She confesses she has trouble meeting new friends and talking at a deeper level with people. But she knew she could call me and I would understand what she was going through. I would listen and I would talk.

"Boy, it's wonderful to find someone who really listens to what I have to say," one new friend says to another. "I wish my husband could communicate like this with me." The other new friend responds by saying: "Yeah, I know what you mean. My wife is so darn busy with her career she hardly gives me the time of day."

The thing is, I think I do understand more than the average man or woman on the street what Sara is going through. "Most people can't fathom what I'm talking about when I tell them I'm afraid to make commitments for fear of having to back out," she says over the phone. "You know what I'm talking about." She asks for advice on how to crawl out of the pit of depression and get excited again about her part-time career. I become part consultant, part counselor, part friend and, perhaps, part lover (though not in a physical sense). I suggest some steps she can take to get back in the career groove.

The new friends wake up in their separate beds, in their separate homes, and their first thoughts are of each other. They count the days until their next meeting. They begin to think about what they will say and what they will do when their paths next cross. For the first time since high school, they feel their hearts skip a beat when they see one another – perhaps at the out-of-town restaurant they chose as a rendezvous. They begin to share their individual hopes and dreams, their individual fears and frustrations. They share every detail of themselves with one another, communicating in ways they have not done with their spouses for years. One of the friends shares a poignant story and tears come. Their hands touch, their eyes lock and their hearts intertwine.

I was prone to emotional affairs for the first 20 years of my marriage. I never succumbed to the physical temptation, but did allow my heart and mind to wander to other women. Interestingly, the women I dated before getting married, the women who have attracted me since my wedding, and my long-time wife all share one or two things in common. They all either have health problems or came from troubled childhood homes. These women needed a listening ear and a sensitive heart. I also assumed they needed someone handy who had a "caretaker's" mindset. And boy, did I know how to play that role. Being a "caretaker" is especially easy to play with other women. I could be the part-time co-dependent person in their lives without having to wash their dishes and diaper their babies and pay their bills and perform in their beds. They saw me at my public best rather than in those nasty times of reality when I screamed at the kids or woke up with matted hair or became old and grumpy paying bills.

The friends become lovers because of their communication rather than their looks. Covert lunch dates between new friends is one thing, but lovers need more than that. He tells his wife about an important business meeting in Des Moines. She tells her husband about getting together with an old high-school friend in Iowa City. The two friends physically consummate their relationship and become secret lovers. They prove the myth wrong.

"You need to set some small, bite-sized goals for yourself, Sara," I say into the phone. *"Don't try to go for the whole shebang at once. Work yourself back into professional shape. The most important thing, though, is to find a few close friends to talk to." There is a pause. "And I can't play that role." Another pause. "I know you can't," she says. We hung up a minute later and I get ready to leave the office and head for home. There is a small part of me, however, that wants to call Sara back, find out her address, visit her in person and let her spill her guts. I could give her comforting words.*

Instead, I go home, partially because I refuse to again put on the label of "caretaker" – for Sherrie, Sara or anyone. Mainly, however, I go home because I love Sherrie more than anything and anyone else in the world.

A Wimpy Villain

— *or* —

The Puppy Play: A Tragedy

Sherrie walked toward me in the backyard while I picked up dog poop. I don't particularly like pooper-scooper duty. If I'm totally honest, I don't really like dogs that much either, unless they are running free on some expansive farm or ranch.

"I reaalllly reaallly want to ask you something," Sherrie said while doing an impassioned impersonation of a fairy-tale damsel in distress. Actually, she had been in distress – after recently having returned from the hospital where she underwent another surgery (unrelated to fibromyalgia).

"I want, no, I need another dog," she said. "I want a puppy I can cuddle and train." Evidently, one old dog was not sufficient to fulfill her cuddle quotient. I dropped my dog-poop tools and crossed my arms. Sherrie knew I found her request as disgusting as my backyard assignment.

Interlude – I know many of you readers think I'm a poop head right about now. How can I deny a recent hospital patient a tail-wagging puppy? Some of you assume I must be Cruella Deville's evil stepson who just stepped off the set of "101 Dalmatians." C'mon, Piburn, have a heart. The loved one needs to support the person with a chronic condition. True, support is important in a relationship slapped silly by chronic illness. But to what degree, and at what cost? And where do truth and openness come into play?

Sherrie said: "I know we've had major problems with dogs in the past . . . but this time it will be different." I thought: It will be the same as always.

Sherrie said: "I'll get up with it in the night if it whines and pick up the poop in the yard." I thought: Only at first and then I'll become the designated puppy "caretaker," which, in my case, means becoming a cranky canine caregiver.

Sherrie said: "The kids will help if I can't do it." I thought: Give . . . me . . . a . . . break. Do you have another litter of kids I don't know about that likes doing chores?

Sherrie said: "This time, I'll really train the dog the right way." I thought: If you were well, that might happen. With your fatigue and bad back, I don't think so.

Sherrie said: "Can I start looking for a puppy?" I said: "Sure." But I'm thinking something that's not fit to print in a book published for public consumption.

Two days later, DG joined the clan. Sherrie and the kids loved the novelty of having a mixed-labrador puppy roaming the house. I disliked the regular routine of finding puppy poop on the carpet. Speaking again of poop, I felt pooped. While Sherrie was in the hospital, I had kept a hundred parental and professional concerns on course. Sherrie and I both needed many good nights of catch-up sleep. DG, on the other hand, was ready to roll each morning at 4:30. The first few mornings Sherrie got up to take care of DG, who refused to go back in her crate once she awakened. But I saw how much that took out of Sherrie. So I played the good, stoical soldier and got up the next several mornings. I played the unwritten script everyone knew I would.

The cute puppy brought out my meanness. My words and actions became cutting to everything and everybody involved with the puppy. I said "sure" when Sherrie asked if she could have a puppy, but I intended to make everyone emotionally and mentally pay for my perceived magnanimity. The tangible little dog came to symbolize all that I hated about chronic illness. A month or so after DG arrived, Sherrie unexpectedly returned to the hospital for several days. During that stint I had to keep parenting, professional and puppy plates spinning at the same time. The puppy was the straw that broke my back. Her wee-hour wailing drove me to the verge of killing her. I called Sherrie at the hospital and confessed I was considering ending the dog's natural life. She knew I wasn't kidding and I was thankful Sherrie called a friend of hers who was willing to watch DG for the remainder of her hospital stay.

DG came home a day after Sherrie returned and the next seven days were miserable for everyone, including the puppy. Everything about our lives seemed out of control. Except for Bret, a toddler then, family members decided DG had to go. The next day, I made the dreaded trek, with the unsuspecting puppy, to the Humane Society. Unfortunately, we have returned two or three Piburn dogs to that organization over the years. I hope they all found good homes with merciful masters. They might have also made a quick exit to "doggie heaven."

So, you see, "The Puppy Play" is a tragedy. And who is the villain? Why, of course, it is me. But I'm not the villain because

I dislike dogs, or because I considered "mutt murder" or because I drove the animal back to the pound. The villainous act was in the kind-hearted way I said, "Sure." By refusing to say what I thought in that backyard conversation, I set in motion the whole twisted plot. My wimpy "sure" was more damaging than a simple "no." My ongoing meanness belittled Sherrie, the puppy, my family and the truth. Society tells "caretakers" to be nice. Our politeness is often the cause of discontent.

SECTION TWO ACTION PAGE:

Tap Into the Feelings

1. Write a hole-in-the-wall letter

Get out of your nice and polite "caretaker" mindset. Forget all the "shoulds" and "should nots" you have learned in life. For a few minutes, be like the acerbic dragon slayer who threatens to punch out a dim-witted doctor or the prehistoric cave dweller who punches a hole in the wall. But instead of screaming or throwing a left hook, you just need to write a letter. Think about something or someone that really makes you angry. Maybe it is a health-insurance claims adjuster or a sassy baby-sitter or the monthly medical bills. Write that person or thing a letter – a nasty one. Don't hold back. Let the emotions and words spew as if from a volcano. You don't give a hoot about correct punctuation or grammar. You are letting the words flow freely and quickly from deep within your gut. Try to fill up at least a page and do it within five minutes.

After you finish writing the letter, take a five-minute break. Then come back and read the letter over. One result might be that your anger has subsided. The process of writing the letter was akin to the steam let off by a pressure cooker; it prevents a major explosion. Another result is you will decide, after checking your motive, that you need to communicate with the person you wrote. Decide upon a plan that allows you to get your points across without verbally or physically hurting the person to whom your anger is directed. This activity ends by tearing up the letter and throwing it away. That does not mean your words were worthless. It does symbolize, however, that the letter is only a means to an end, not an end in itself.

2. Conduct a personal puppy patrol

What is the "unwanted puppy" in your life that you are not being truthful about? Is it a vacation others want you to take? Is it a job relocation you have hesitantly accepted? In your notebook, write the answers to the following questions.

A. In a word or phrase, who or what is the "unwanted puppy" in your life?
B. Who, if anyone, is forcing you to accept that "puppy"?
C. In your heart of hearts, what would you prefer to do regarding the "puppy"?
D. Why have you accepted the "puppy" so far?
E. What would be the ramifications of pushing for "C," instead of accepting "A"?
F. What steps could you take to break out of the pseudo-community phase in hopes of achieving "C"?
G. Finish reading this entire book, then go back and revise "F," if need be.
H. Put "C" into action.

3. Learn from "The Fat Lady"

On a sheet of paper, list what "The Fat Lady" of chronic illness has taught you about yourself and your chronically ill loved one. How can you use those lessons learned to improve one or two areas of your life?

4. Mine for gold

Out of all the essays and suggested activities in this section, what do you believe is the most significant and/or memorable nugget for you?

_____

_____

_____

• What is the "first step" you will take toward making that nugget truly impact your life for the better?

• I will_____ (what?)

by _____ (when?)

EXAMPLE: I will, by the end of the month, suggest that our chronic illness support group offer a program to help "partners" sometime in the next three months and on a periodic basis thereafter.

RAISE THE
WHITE FLAG

phase three

Emptiness. Populated by vulnerable people. Epitomized by vulnerability, honesty, human connections.

"*I'm done playing charades; please help me.*"

chapter 7

LOOKING
INWARD

Introspection can be an important step on the
path of personal growth.

Truth & Courage

— *or* —

The Flashing Oil Light

Let's say the open road calls my name and I bolt, feeling the freedom of a cheetah racing across the Serengeti as I put the pedal to the metal. The white lines of a two-lane prairie highway flash and disappear outside the driver's window. I lose track of time. The black canvas of night fills my windshield and then snow falls like feathers burst from a pillow. Then, let's say, I realize I haven't a clue where I am other than in the midst of a blizzard. My car and I are the only moving things on this isolated road. At midnight the oil light on the car's dashboard comes on. Time out.

Question: Is it good or bad that the oil light flashes? Most people respond to that question with an emphatic, "Bad!" Let's reconsider that for a minute. It's as if a little mechanic lives underneath the hood of my car. He checks all the gauges and mechanical parts and lets me know when things need attention. "Oops, the car needs oil," the mechanic says to himself. "I'll let Piburn know." The oil light flashes. The mechanic gives me information to help me negotiate this bitter slice of life. That flashing light is his way of saying, "I thought you should know that the car is low on oil. I'm not telling you what to do about it. I just wanted to give you some important data so you can make the best decision."

My answer to the question: The flashing oil light is neither good nor bad, it just is. The flashing oil light represents another data point for me to consider in the midst of that particular situation. True, I would prefer not being low on oil, but since that is the case, I appreciate knowing about it.

The scene switches to another dashboard – this one in my heart. A tiny woman (gender bias again) sits at the control panel of my emotions. She presses a button that lights up to tell me something such as, "You're angry." Most of us have grown up assuming there are good feelings – happiness, excitement, peacefulness – and bad feelings – madness, sadness, fear. We learned those lessons early on. "You're angry, go to your room." "Big boys don't cry." Message: Being mad or sad is bad, worthy of punishment or ridicule.

Those early lessons sentenced many people to life behind emotional bars. Their fear of their own feelings keeps them trapped. They can't admit they are angry or fearful because those feelings are bad. Hell, they might think that to be mad or sad means they themselves are bad. The kind little woman at the control panel means nothing of the sort. Like her mechanic counterpart, she is merely providing data. "Gregg," she says with her flashing light, "you're angry. I'm not telling you what to do about that. I just thought you would appreciate having that extra information."

Most often I would prefer not to be angry, but if that's the case, I'm glad to know about it. True, I normally prefer Sherrie (or other loved ones) not to be mad, but if she is, I'm glad to know about it. The powerful lesson that contradicts those early lessons is that emotions are neither right nor wrong, they just are. This simple phrase can revolutionize your life. It means you don't have to hold it all in. The rules have changed. Big boys can cry. It's healthy and relaxing to do so. The new rules give you permission to feel mad or scared or nervous or depressed. These rules also say it's OK for you to share your feelings. You are providing data, not committing or confessing to a mortal sin.

The early lessons shaped us into upright pressure cookers with all the vents closed. If you hold all those emotions in, eventually you're going to create an explosive outburst. If you've held those feelings in a long time, the outburst is likely to be quite spicy, leading you to say things that will severely hurt your loved ones. That is when your verbal response to your emotions turns bad or even catastrophic, as in the chaos of phase two.

In a relationship staggering under the weight of chronic illness, the freedom to share feelings is crucial. Of course such a philosophy is a wallop upside the head of the "caretaker's" job description, which states you must be an unfeeling rock, the John Wayne of support, the Robotron of Efficiency. We think that by stifling our emotions we are helping our loved one who is ill, but we are living a lie and being unfair by keeping important information from that person.

My stoicism is my lie. I fear admitting fear. What will she think of me? How will she respect me? Why would she continue to love me?

At long last, through trial and error, I began sharing my emotions, my fears. Amazingly, because of that, Sherrie thinks more highly of me now. She seems to respect my actions more than ever. I know, through her words and touch, that her love for me grows as my openness and honesty grow. Then it dawns on me. In this culture it takes courage to appropriately convey true feelings. It is the true courage pseudo-community "caretakers" only dream about.

Oh, we silent, macho types make fun of "sensitive New Age guys" but our sarcasm masks our fear of being honest. To tell it like it is, including an explanation of your feelings, takes guts. It makes sense Sherrie would love me more when I combine truth and courage – a powerful and attractive one-two punch in the love game.

My fear, my sadness, my joy and my anger are neither right nor wrong; they just are. It is another data point to living with a loved one who happens to be chronically ill. And my fear, when expressed openly and appropriately, is truth. As historian Ken Burns says, "If it has no emotion, it has no meaning." We rob our discussions and relationships of huge chunks of meaning by leaving the heart side of the equation blank.

Chronic illness darkens our present and future. Living by the old lessons, living the life of a pressure cooker, is akin to putting on sunglasses at night. It turns an already bleak situation bleaker. Telling the truth and sharing your feelings are ways to bring light to darkness, turn grief into growth, change constant challenge into greater love, stoicism into courage.

Journal to the Center of Yourself

— or —

Getting an Emotional Jump-Start

*"If dentists were psychologists I would call the night number
and report I'm suffering from an emotional dry socket."*
– Gregg Piburn, Journal excerpt: Oct. 10, 1989

The "caretaker" profile calls for us to suck it up, keep a stiff
upper lip, carry the weight of the world on our shoul-
ders, while all the time being as wholesome and competent as
Clara Barton, nurse extraordinaire and founder of the Red
Cross. Obviously, I encourage readers to take a different path.
Daniel Goleman published a book in 1995 titled, *Emotional
Intelligence: Why it can Matter More than IQ.* Among many
other things, he had this to say about emotional intelligence:

"Much evidence testifies that people who are
emotionally adept – who know and manage their
own feelings well, and who read and deal effectively
with other people's feelings – are at an advantage in
any domain of life, whether romance and intimate
relationships or picking up the unspoken rules
that govern success in organizational politics. People with well-developed emotional skills are also
more likely to be content and effective in their lives,
mastering the habits of mind that foster their own

productivity; people who cannot marshal some control over their emotional life fight inner battles that sabotage their ability for focused work and clear thought."

The suck-it-up approach to handling chronic illness definitely goes contrary to Goleman's advice.

"The male beast is . . . well, a dumb beast for the most part. We don't listen, we don't talk, we don't feel, we don't live. We present, we analyze, we play the angles, we work."
— Journal excerpt: Jan. 27, 1988

I grew up in the 1950s and watched more episodes of "The Lone Ranger" and "Bonanza," among many other westerns, than I care to consider. My TV heroes had a low emotional quotient (EQ). When Sherrie got sick in the mid-'80s, my EQ was a nice, round number – 0. I believe I have a high EQ now, thanks in large part to Sherrie's sometimes gentle, sometimes stern coaching. One other factor that helped me raise my EQ was writing more than 3,000 journal entries during a decade of Sherrie's illness.

"Yes, I still have dreams, sweet wife of my youth, but I've let the grind of life slowly steam roll them into some unrecognizable road kill."
— Journal excerpt: Dec. 28, 1989

The journal invited me to spill my guts. It taught me to recognize the feelings I had always kept buried and helped me work through many problems. The journal figuratively offered a listening ear when I still feared telling others what was going on in my head and heart. Writing journal entries was akin to spending several days on the beginner's ski slope, getting a feel for the boards on my feet. I was not ready to leap onto the emotional chair lift and shoot down the steep runs designed for experts. The journal helped me get the feel of my emotions.

"I feel as if a crazed penitentiary warden has drawn the curtains of my cell window, shown me the bright light of life's potential, let me smell the aroma of boundless joy, and opened the heavy, iron doors so I could take my first tentative steps toward freedom, only to have his uniformed thugs hurl me back into my cage as their insidious guffaws echo through the chambers."
— *Journal excerpt: Sept. 18, 1991*

The following suggestions coincide with how I approached journal writing. However, a journal is extremely personal so you might develop your own philosophy and approach.

1. Do not worry about spelling or grammar. Let the words spill out from your mind and heart onto the printed page or computer screen. This is an exercise in getting in touch with your emotions, not a writing assignment from your stern seventh-grade English teacher.
2. Focus on one or two thoughts per entry. A diary documents events and activities. A journal delves into insights and wisdom. Be attentive to the sights and sounds around you that might spark a new thought. I have written entire entries based on one phrase I happened to overhear or one sighting of a bird in flight.

"If chronic illness had a face, it would be pockmarked and sporting a devilish expression, perhaps with a tinge of yellow glowing from its eye sockets."
— *Journal excerpt: Sept. 22, 1991*

3. Write every day. This is especially important for those who struggle with writing. The more you do it, the easier it becomes. For some, scheduling a certain part of each day for writing will help you stay on track.

4. Choose a format that works best for you. My notebook computer is an important tool of my trade. It made sense for me to use the computer to write the entries, and print them out on paper, before placing them into three-ringed binders. A Big Chief Tablet, however, is just as valid a choice for your journal.

5. Enjoy the process. If the journal is a drag, you are not doing something right. This is a chance to get to know yourself better. It is a worthwhile venture and should be cause for joy.

"Not always, but sometimes a new day is like a clean slate. Yesterday afternoon and evening were quite horrid. But today I feel as if yesterday's problems are ancient history and that we can move forward as a family and I can go on as a man."
— *Journal excerpt: March 10, 1995*

6. Be creative. Sometimes my entries are letters to God. Sometimes one of my personalities (Lance the Adventurer) writes a letter to another part of me (Walter the Accountant). I have even written to dead relatives and then, perhaps a day later, I assumed the role of the dead relative and wrote myself a reply.

One day you might feel like writing a poem. Another day you might simply draw a picture. Vary the action to keep the journal alive.

7. Periodically read past entries. For many years I read two entries daily from previous years. For example, on May 2, 1995, I read my entries from May 2, 1994, and May 2, 1991. You will sense trends in your life, see that some issues continue to hold you back, and discover you resolved some old problems.

"The past six weeks has sucked the adrenaline from my body – like a vampire sucking my blood. At 9:30 I had hoped to crash because I felt exhausted from the past several days. Now, I have ventured into a realm beyond tired, feeling as if I crashed into an emotional brick wall.
— Journal excerpt: March 18, 1993

I do have one warning, however. If the journal becomes your only confidant, that is unhealthy. Several months ago I stopped writing daily journal entries (I still do them occasionally) and found myself talking more to Sherrie, my kids and my close friends. I frequently remind myself to tell people things I used to save only for the journal. I needed the journal to provide a jump-start for my rising emotional intelligence. Now I'm able and willing to tell my loved ones what is on my mind and in my heart.

At first my emotions were stuck in my heart. Then the journal helped me get them into my brain and onto paper. Now my feelings can travel directly from my heart to those whom I love.

"Seven things I fear, one I despise:
A life of empty words
A goal without power
A mission denied
A final farewell
A loneliness strong
A face without laughter
A soul without song"

— *Journal excerpt: May 14, 1991*

Author Alfred Kazin said, "In a real sense, the writer writes in order to teach himself." In a real sense, both an author and a journal writer reap this same reward.

Empty in St. Louis

— or —

Twelve Men Out of the Comfort Zone

Twelve male managers from a nationwide manufacturing company sat in a semi-circle waiting for me to lead them through a day-long retreat. Executives from across the country had converged at our meeting in St. Louis. This seemed to be a group that wanted to get down to business from the get-go. The only constant element of my retreats is introducing groups to the four phases in the morning workshop sessions, which creates the kind of open, honest and courageous environment needed to make our work relevant and memorable. This was the first time the top managers had met since a beloved president of their company had died six months earlier.

In the afternoon, each manager gave a 15-minute report on the accomplishments of the past six months and the plans they had for the rest of the year. The new president (I'll call him Joe) had been a top manager with the company for several years. He gave a wrap-up report. It went sort of like this:

"This has been a great day. I've been pretty nervous about getting you all together since this is my first meeting as president. I can't tell you how much I appreciate having you all on my team." He paused, then tears came to the corners of his eyes. "What you have been doing the last six months is great." He paused again, catching his breath. "I appreciate your efforts very much. But I appreciate your support since I took over as president even more. It's been hard, taking over from Bob." The president's lower lip started to quiver. "I know everyone in this room loved him and misses him. I know I sure do." Tears trickled down his cheeks and his voice caught. The hotel meeting room itself seemed to hold its breath a few seconds. Then, with quivering voice, the president looked at me and said, "I can't go on. That's all I can say."

He sat down, and I waited to see what would happen. As I expected, it didn't take long for someone to come to the rescue. "Uh, Joe," the company comptroller said to the president after four seconds of silence, "give us an update on that new training program we're developing."

The president had already regained his composure and started to give an update. I let his update last, oh, about five seconds before I interrupted. "What just happened regarding the four phases?" I said. A young manager said, "We went from phase one to phase three and back to phase one in about five seconds." I replied, "You got it. So do you guys want to stay in pseudo-community and let Joe finish his training pro gram update or do you want to see what emptiness is really like?" Again, silence. But this time it was followed a few seconds later by another manager saying, "Let's delve into phase three." I saw three or four heads nod up and down and I figured that was enough of a mandate to go for it.

I had each manager respond to the president's 30-second speech as well as comment on anything else they wanted. It took 45 minutes to go around the room. Some amazing thoughts and feelings came out from this hairy-knuckled group. They were able to publicly grieve over the loss of their beloved leader, while also thank their new president for his efforts during a difficult time for the company. A manager who had been with the company for many years said, "Joe, I always knew you were a capable manager, but I wasn't sure how much you cared about the company and its employees. Now I know how much you care. I'm ready and willing to support you any way I can."

In the pseudo-community phase, the president's 30-second speech would have been an embarrassment. Because people caught in phase one pretend life is easy. It might be a career-limiting error to show vulnerability. A group that delves into emptiness knows life is difficult and that it takes a strong person to show vulnerability. I told Joe after the meeting that he will likely never give a more powerful and meaningful speech.

Remember, an invisible barbed-wire fence separates phases one and two from phases three and four. Joe's unbridled emotions drove the whole group through that barbed wire, but the natural inclination to get back into a comfort zone quickly dragged the group back to the pseudo-community phase. They needed a nudge from me to go back to the higher realm of group interaction.

So what does this business anecdote have to do with chronic illness? A whole lot, because it illustrates the power of being vulnerable and of "turning on the lights" to heart-felt, open communication. If 12 male managers born in the 1940s and 1950s can communicate beyond the barbed wire, then you and your chronically-ill loved one should be able to, also. Once you spend time beyond the confines of phases one and two, you will never want to go back to those limiting and untruthful environments. Take a risk and bust through "the barbed wire." Your relationship will never be the same.

Dealing with Denial

— *or* —

A Losses List

I saw an acquaintance in the lobby at the local movie theater. We engaged in idle chit-chat while I waited for Sherrie to come out of the rest room. Then he said, "My wife has had diabetes now for about a year."

"Oh, I'm sorry," I said. "How are you doing with that?" He quickly smiled and said: "Oh, I'm fine. Sally is doing well, too. It's not a biggie at all. Life goes on."

Let's probe his response for a minute. For one thing, he might just be "clipping the question" as I suggested doing with acquaintances in an essay in the previous chapter. If so, his answer was fine. However, I sensed what he said to me was likely similar to what he says to his parents, his closest friends, or his wife. Some of you might believe his answer represented a positive attitude that will help he and his wife overcome problems associated with her illness. Perhaps you are right, but I believe such an overriding positive attitude could be denial in disguise.

Back in the days when I dwelled in denial, I often used a phrase I learned as a kid. "Oh, it could always be worse." It's one of those phrases that, although true, can belittle the situation and the people involved. Yes, Sherrie went in for back surgeries rather than cancer surgeries. Yes, Sherrie has been ill, but all our children have been healthy. Yes, Sherrie is still alive while one of our good friends has been dead for 25 years thanks to a drunk driver.

Yes, it could be worse . . . and it could be better.

For me, it became important to begin grieving our losses caused by "The Intruder." As most people know, the grief process mandates the need to tap into the emotions that arise from loss. However, many people believe the grief process relates only to the death of a loved one. In fact, it's healthy to grieve any significant loss. As a way of helping readers break through "the barbed wire" into emptiness, I am going to list some of the losses Sherrie and I felt since she became ill in 1985. When you get to the action page at the end of section three, you will have a chance to do the same thing.

LOSSES CAUSED PRIMARILY OR TOTALLY BY SHERRIE'S CHRONIC CONDITIONS

• **Recreational opportunities** – We can't go backpacking or skiing, for example, as a couple or as a family.

• **Income** – Being a single-income family nowadays is a challenge, especially when high medical costs get thrown into the equation. Before Sherrie started feeling so bad, she was able to work part-time; now that income is gone as well.

• **A fine house and good neighborhood** – We moved to a bigger, much more expensive house because everything Sherrie needs is on one floor. This might sound as if it's a win rather than a loss, but had Sherrie not been injured in a car accident, resulting in chronic back problems, we could have stayed in a house we liked without adding huge expenses to our budget.

• **Friendships** – Some of our friends from the old, healthy days could not handle changes brought on by Sherrie's illness. They got miffed when we occasionally canceled plans with them because Sherrie felt horrid. We drifted apart, and we rarely, if ever, see them anymore.

• **Self-esteem** – In her eyes, Sherrie became a homemaker who often could not do the duties of a homemaker. Sadly, she found many of her peers pooh-poohed "mere homemakers." Where did that leave her self-esteem? During the worst times, she became a "patient" whose illness defined her identity.

• **Envisioned motherhood** – While Corlet swam in the womb, Sherrie and I talked about becoming parents. Sherrie longed to be an active mother who would eventually go on long hikes with her children, teach them how to ski, show them the ropes of how to camp in the Rockies and model the joys of a physically active life. Chronic illness eliminated that vision while Corlet was a toddler and Alyse an infant.

• **Dreams** – Like many young couples, Sherrie and I talked for hours about what our lives together would be like. None of those dreams included visions of hospital stays or operations or exhaustion or defeat or depression.

• **Freedom** – At times Sherrie's poor health caused us to cancel vacation plans at the last minute, sit at home alone during the holidays instead of spending time with extended family, and decline invitations to try new activities such as water skiing, among other things. Chronic illness constructs visible and invisible barriers around your life, making you sometimes feel as trapped as a ward of the state.

These are a few losses we have felt thanks to chronic illness. I do not, repeat, do NOT suggest you dwell on your losses. But I do believe there is value in naming the losses so that you can tap into those restrained emotions and break out of the pseudo-community and chaos phases. Without naming the losses, you might fool yourself into believing chronic illness is nothing more than a minor nuisance. We don't typically adapt our lives significantly in reaction to minor nuisances. We just keep plodding through life as we always did.

Once Sherrie and I knew we were battling a significant enemy, we eventually came to the conclusion that we needed to discuss our losses and adapt our lives. We had to reassess our careers, develop new friendships, evaluate our parenting and create new dreams. We might have kept plodding along had we chosen the comfort and denial of pseudo-community rather than the temporary discomfort of assessing our losses.

Obviously, you must become vulnerable to think and speak about losses. Those who operate in phases one and two believe vulnerable people are weak people. I believe the opposite is true. Show me people who refuse to let their guard down and I'll show you individuals who are unsure of themselves and lack the courage to be real. Vulnerable people are strong people.

What losses have you felt because of chronic illness? Talk about them to people you can trust. Feel the emotions brought on by those losses. Then decide what you can learn from them and do about them. This process might take weeks or months, but it is a valuable investment of time and energy. Turn on the lights through open, honest and courageous communication and make some adjustments (which means taking back control of your lives).

It's easier to fight a foe who is out in the open rather than one that is hidden in the jungle of the mind. It's important to know that you and a loved one are adjusting to your life with chronic illness together, not separately. Count your losses, make adjustments and revel in building a new and deeper relationship beyond the confines of "the barbed wire."

Cutting Our Losses

— *or* —

A Little Madness

Alyse and I drove to the end of the dirt lane that stands above Moose Pond. I wanted to say good-bye to Bret, who was playing with a homemade whip.

"Hey, my little man, we're heading back to Loveland," I said, stroking the back of his curly-haired head.

"OK, Dad," he said.

"I'm going to miss you for the next few days but I'm sure glad you and Sherrie get to spend time up at the cabin."

"Me, too."

Then Alyse slowly drove the car away from her brother, my son, one of my three special joys in the world. If you recall, I am Corlet and Alyse's biological father, but Sherrie and I adopted Bret when he was three days old. I glanced into the rearview mirror and saw Bret walk back toward the pond, toward some new boyhood adventure. And I felt a lump in my throat, knowing how much I've come to depend on his presence for my happiness.

The previous essay spoke about losses caused by Sherrie's illnesses. In 1987, she had a hysterectomy, which produced yet another loss – the potential of conceiving a third child. I felt OK about that, believing that bringing two children into this volatile world is enough. Sherrie, on the other hand, still felt a hole in her spirit, a cavity that could only be filled by becoming the mother of one more child, a son. It took me a while to share that vision, already feeling overwhelmed by my personal and professional duties. But I finally came to the conclusion that adopting a son could put a final exclamation point to our nuclear family.

We started the adoption process through an organization that specialized in international matches. Even though Sherrie's fibromyalgia symptoms sometimes flattened her for a week at a time, we convinced ourselves we could manage a third child. Naturally, some others who knew our situation thought we were insane. We began to wonder ourselves if we were loony when Sherrie's back started hurting. Doctors guessed her problems came from many years of an overly active life, which included teaching hours and hours of aerobics classes as part of her pre-illness career. Finally, on Jan. 26, 1988, she went in for a laminectomy. Unfortunately, the back surgery did not clear up her problems. Sherrie felt back pain almost constantly, and we again wondered about the logic of bringing a baby into the family.

After many rational discussions about our options, we agreed on a strategy. In September 1988 I wrote a letter to the agency saying we still wanted to adopt a child. But because of Sherrie's surgery and ongoing problems, we asked them not to honor our request for six months. At the end of that time, I added, we would contact the agency to say whether we wanted to bow out of the program or continue with the process. There, that was settled. Now Sherrie could focus on getting better and we would not have the added anxiety of wading through the adoption process. The universe, of course, doesn't pay much attention to silly little plans created by mere mortals. About three weeks later, on Oct. 6, 1988, Sherrie got a call while I was at K-Mart getting paint for the kitchen walls. When I got back, she said we had to talk. This is how I described our conversation in my journal entry for that day.

"Sherrie got Alyse set up in front of the television and asked me to follow her into the bedroom. The look on her face communicated that she had some important news for me. I assumed somebody had died. Her next words were startling: 'The agency called and they have a baby for us.'

"Not only was I shocked, I was surprisingly thrilled. Deep down I was happy about the prospect of having a son, but I knew there was a good reason we had decided to put that decision on hold. This morning I discovered it is much easier to say 'wait' to a concept (adoption) than 'no' to a specific baby."

I learned more about the situation as Sherrie continued to tell me about the phone conversation she had earlier in the day. The baby we wanted had been born the day before and his mother was a Colorado teenager. They needed an answer quickly. We decided to ask if we could think it over for a day. On Oct. 7 we called to tell the agency we wanted to travel the 100 miles or so the next day to talk to agency officials and maybe, just maybe, take a peek at the baby. On Oct. 8 we drove to the agency with the intention of checking out the situation. In our heart of hearts, however, we both knew we would be bringing home a son. We slipped an old car seat and our daughters' Cabbage Patch Doll clothes into the car.

When we saw the bald-headed little boy we fell in love with him. I called my parents and, after telling Mom the news, asked her to put Alyse and Corlet on the line.

"We're bringing home a little brother for you," I said. They went nuts.

"How old is he?" Corlet asked.

"Three days," I said.

"What's his name?" Alyse asked.

"Remember, we talked about naming him Bret."

"Gramma, his name is Bret and he's three days old!" I heard Corlet scream.

But, as with all real stories, the road has been rough and wild having three children. I confess there have been a few days along the way when I wondered about the sanity of adding a third child to our family. (For those of you with three or more children, you likely understand that generally the group dynamics of having three children is much more complex than having two.) Were we crazy to add another child to our clan in the midst of Sherrie's chronic illness and pain? Ab-so-lute-ly. On Aug. 14, 1989, Sherrie had a lower-back fusion to help relieve her pain. For the next few months she refrained from lifting anything more than five pounds. Bret was less than a year old and not yet walking during the first stage of Sherrie's recovery. Yet somehow we managed.

Were we really crazy? No doubt about it. It was ludicrous to bring a third child into our family under the circumstances. We were a family who had already survived many losses and had no business pretending we could handle a newborn. And as most parents realize, the issues change, but challenges remain at every stage of a child's life. So, were we crazy? You betcha. But for whatever reason, the Piburns needed to be a family of five, rather than four.

Nikos Kazantakis wrote a book titled, *Zorba the Greek*. In one passage, Zorba says: "Boss, you've got everything except one thing – madness! A man needs a little madness or else he never dares cut the rope to be free."

Chronic illness felt like chains in some areas of our lives. One of those areas seemed to be the size of our family. We decided we did not want chronic illness to have the final say in something so important. The trick is determining when to avoid the madness and when to dive into the center of its core. Yes, we were crazy, filled with madness. And today I am free to love a boy who magically came into our lives despite all the reasons he shouldn't have. Chronic illness sprouts madness in a family. And we don't regret that we got a little bit crazy, especially when the result of our madness is a life-long relationship with a beloved young boy, our son.

1992: Part 1

— *or* —

Grief & Growth

On Aug. 3, 1993, I had breakfast with a former boss. We had not seen each other for a year. She asked, "So how was 1992 for you?" I paused for a few seconds, trying to put a million emotions and thoughts into one statement. I replied, "1992 was a year of grief and growth." This essay and the next reveal some of those thoughts and feelings as written in my journal during 1992. I also jotted down additional thoughts from the perspective of later years.

"Dear Lord: Maybe what I am feeling this Jan. 1 is a divine dissatisfaction with life, a concern that drives me toward self-improvement rather than self-pity. Lord, may I be real in a real weird world in 1992."
— Journal excerpt: Jan. 1, 1992.

The five of us were floating with life jackets in an underground river at Xcaret, a natural-environment amusement park 90 minutes south of Cancun, Mexico. It was spring break 1997. Although it is far from pitch black, the popular river float is almost totally underground. Sometimes you don't have to move a muscle for the current to gently carry you along.

Other times you have to kick and stroke with your legs and arms to move downstream.

"I'm tumbling, rolling over and over in the white, powdery snow, feeling lightheaded for a while, then feeling the white gold turn sticky, heavy, suffocating. It is the excitement of new challenges . . . doing what one loves. Then it gets all fouled up by those who try to add on other things. You say 'yes' once, then twice, then the avalanche is on. Rolling and spinning, ducking and bobbing, until the light of the sun illuminating the blue sky vanishes from sight. It is a white blackness, causing you to wonder where the hell you are and how you are going to dig yourself out of this seductive mess. Then you close your eyes and go to sleep, hoping that while you rest the blanket of death will melt away."
— *Journal entry: Jan. 23, 1992.*

Sometimes chronic illness carries a family along like a river that forces a bottle to go along its course to the prairie. Other times family members have to kick like crazy to just stay above the surface, to just survive chronic illness. All families eventually deal with their own crosses, be it chronic illness or some other difficulty. And for certain seasons of an individual's or family's life, they bear more than one cross.

"I gave a presentation at an addiction seminar this morning and was my typical charismatic self. People laughed, seemingly feeling good about my presence in this place. How gloriously alive and happy I feel when I bring joy to others, even strangers. On the flip side, some 12 hours later, I raced into Bret's bedroom and said, in a gruff voice, 'What do you want, Bret? I told you I

would close the door if I saw your face again today!' Wham!
What a farce. I come across like a cross between Mother Teresa
and Jay Leno to the public and act like a combination Saddam
Hussein and Archie Bunker at home."
— Journal excerpt: Feb. 29, 1992.

In 1992, several of Sherrie's crosses, besides chronic illness, converged on our family.

"When I got home from work, Bret hugged me tightly around
the neck. Sherrie left to take the girls shopping. Twenty minutes
later my buddy Greg called. We were having one of our typical
crazy conversations. The laughter ended for a moment and
Greg said, 'Is Sherrie all right?' Before I could answer he added
that Sherrie had left a message on his answering machine . . .
'and she sounded rather desperate.'"
— Journal excerpt: March 14, 1992.

Who wouldn't be desperate when setbacks followed every
improvement? Chronic illness seemed to weaken its hold on
Sherrie occasionally, only to pull her back tightly against its
massive chest. But months of wisdom and growth, along
with ongoing pain and exhaustion, surrounded the blips of
desperation.

"Lord, I want to go home. I am tired of having to be on for my job
at all times. I am mentally sapped from driving through miles and
miles of freeways in a distant city. I am sick about seeing a friend
renew acquaintances with the bottle. I am sorry to hear that Alyse is
so sad about me being gone 'all the time.' I want to forget everything

and everybody for a few days and just huddle with my family. I want to feel their warm breath on my face and I want to hear their laughter in my ears. I want to let down and soak up the love they have for me and pass on to them the love I have."

— *Journal excerpt: May 21, 1992.*

"My woman leaves every night, pretending to be a nurse in a performance of 'South Pacific,' while her real man is in need of a soothing, cool-washcloth kind of touch from a lover/friend. The kids are bouncing around like boiling peas in a kettle. All I want to do with them at this moment is dash them down a painless drain. Then I want to grab an ice cream cone and stick the frigid end on my forehead."

— *Journal excerpt: July 6, 1992.*

Are chronic illness and other life difficulties evil conspirators in a plot to destroy my family? I'm finding life's real answers are seldom simple. Maybe they are messengers rather than marauders. Perhaps they are not the doorways to oblivion, but to illumination.

"I tucked Corlet and Alyse into bed and went upstairs. Thirty minutes later Corlet screamed for help. I rushed down and she was trembling in her bed, saying she heard whispering in Alyse's room. Corlet admitted a scary mystery she read earlier in the day haunted her thoughts. Both girls slept on the hide-a-bed upstairs. And so ends our 19th wedding anniversary."

— *Journal excerpt: Aug. 19, 1992.*

The vast majority of people with CFS are women. The majority of those women are Type-A personalities – the kind of people who drive themselves to success and have a difficult time relaxing. They become human "doings" rather than human beings in their minds. Is it possible that our spirits rush through life so they don't have to face its tough and uncomfortable issues? For many people, the mind, body and soul stay united in this strategy to keep busy and, thus, stay out of arm's reach of the real villain.

"Here's what I didn't get done this weekend: (1) Clean the house, (2) Go to church, (3) Prepare for next week's seminar, and (4) Mow the lawn. Here's what I did get done this weekend: (1) Use golf clubs to hit tennis balls back and forth between Bret and me, (2) Have Alyse sit on my lap and hug her for a few precious seconds, and (3) Go on a bike ride with Bret and Alyse and get stranded in a rainstorm at, of all places, Sunshine Yogurt."
— Journal excerpt: Aug. 23, 1992.

1992: Part 2

— *or* —

With You for the Journey

In the worst of times my internal pessimist imagines how it could become even worse.

"'I have this feeling,' I told Greg and Cindy while we sat around their kitchen table, 'that Sherrie won't live very long. It might be another 15 or 20 years, who knows, but I have a hard time imagining her living to a ripe old age.' Sherrie holes up in a hospital 15 minutes from home, while I try to struggle with the nightmare of balancing so many damn plates and flashbacks of the last seven years of crap. Instead of saying 'to hell with all the outside demands,' I am up late on a Labor Day night figuring out ways to keep everybody happy. As a good friend told me eons ago, I need to 'cut myself some slack.'"

— Journal excerpt: Sept. 7, 1992.

What if the body rebels against the difficulties of life? Maybe the body thinks to itself: "Whoa, I can't keep this pace up. I know something hidden and mysterious keeps this person pinned to the ground and they don't have a clue what it is. I know the person needs to get out of the rat race and replace the busyness with reflection. But it ain't happening. Hmm, perhaps I can force the person to look deep within for the answer if I break down." The driver can't race through life without a mean machine (or a healthy body).

"We both seem to have the same dream that becomes clearer in our minds. It's the wondrous onset of new life in each of us, a chance to break through old thoughts and tired relationships that have been like handcuffs to our marriage and have kept us from an abundant life. Somehow we have continued to love each other even when we had figuratively tied our hands behind our backs and ventured into each day with a self-imposed handicap. But now, with the release of those old paradigms, I know our lives will take on a new sheen that will be brighter and richer than even those magical first dates."
— *Journal excerpt: Sept. 11, 1992.*

Chronic illness as a messenger. Could it be true, or am I just creating a conceptual euphemism?

"Life played a cruel joke on my mom and her loved ones today. Three days ago she sat on the couch eating McDonald's fries and slurping a milk shake, celebrating the great news from the doctor that 'it looks benign.' Yesterday he called back to say the pathologist's report indicated the growth is malignant. My mom has cancer. Shit."
— *Journal excerpt: Oct. 3, 1992.*

Events often remind me of M. Scott Peck's "Life is difficult" statement that begins his classic best-seller, *The Road Less Traveled.* Peck warns that people who believe life is easy often become paralyzed by problems as they cuss the gods or fate.

They wait for their luck to change. They blame others for screwing up life's nice, easy system. They refuse to do anything tangible to resolve the problem.

"'I knew some tragedy was coming in the movie and I kept wondering if the new scene would be where it happened,' Sher said between sobs. 'I feel like my life is like that.' We had just seen 'A River Runs Through It,' a gorgeous movie about the sometimes hideous results of alcoholism on families. 'I sometimes wish I had remained single and childless because I feel like such a burden to everyone,' she said while we sat in the theater parking lot. 'Bullshit!' I said. 'I would be a blithering wimp without you. Seeing you fight the good fight makes me stronger. Besides, I love you and need you.' We both cried for a minute or so, then we drove off into the next pages of our life story."
— *Journal excerpt: Nov. 27, 1992.*

In my childhood daydreams, I glamorized what I thought were easy career pursuits – being a star athlete because of natural ability rather than hard work, being a successful novelist who could crank out books quickly and painlessly rather than as a craftsman. I now understand the richness and grace of one who keeps plugging along, doing his or her best in the face of hardship or heartache, who seeks simple pleasures and victories, who continues life's journey even if the thorn never comes dislodged. I married such a person, such a fighter. She continues the journey despite the cliffs and chasms of chronic illness. But it is not easy for any of us, especially Sherrie, who faces a daily menu of pain, exhaustion and anguish.

"Late last night I asked Sherrie this question: 'So are you going to stick with this family or are you considering bugging out?' With a face that looked frozen in time, mummified if you will, Sherrie maintained a long silence, eyes cast downward. 'I don't know,' she said in a hoarse whisper. 'I might stay . . . and I might bug out.'"

— Journal excerpt: Dec. 11, 1992.

"For years I wondered in a morbid fantasy what it would be like to become a widower or be abandoned in the middle of the night by a distraught spouse. Now I have a hint of what it would be like – a big syringe thrust into your heart that sucks all the lifeblood from the organs and leaves just an empty, raw cavity. The fantasy is a nightmare that has taken on an eerie sense of possibility."

— Journal excerpt: Dec. 13, 1992.

Sherrie and I sat in a circle on the floor with some people who were dealing with a variety of tough issues. It was December 1992. At the end of the session, the counselor asked everyone to say one "laser statement" that described the essence of their feelings and learnings for the day.

"John, an Andre Agassi look-alike, had trouble coming up with a laser statement and was the last to enter the circle. Finally, when his turn came, he said, 'I now know I deserve to be treated better in this life.' Other statements, in their own ways, were just as powerful. And what was mine? I looked at Sherrie and said, with the group listening in: 'This past year has been a time

of grief and growth. I'm with you for the journey.' Tears came to her eyes."

— *Journal excerpt: Dec. 20, 1992.*

About three of four marriages fail if one of the partners is chronically ill. I imagine the failure rate is even higher if you also throw other significant issues into the equation. Sherrie did not bug out as she thought she might and neither did I. 1992 was our marital "Valley of the Shadow of Death." It was not our last tough year. But because of the rigors of 1992, we have overcome other tough periods and will be able to navigate through future valleys successfully. I'm with you for the journey, Sherrie.

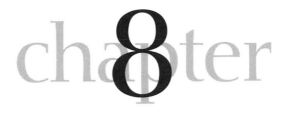

THE "BIG 5" IN PHASE THREE

In the following essays you will see the power of awareness and how it helps you deal with problems in your life.

Support:
Gun Down John Wayne

— *or* —

Tap Into an "Angel"

A year into Sherrie's illness, I was minding my own business on yet another uneventful day in the corporate world. At 11 a.m. the phone on my desk rang. "Gregg, this is Sherilyn. Steve and I want to eat lunch with you in the cafeteria." Others could say those words and they would come out as a request. Sherilyn's words were like a quiet command from Gen. Colin Powell. "Uh, sure, when should we meet?" Steve was a mechanical engineer with the company I worked for. His wife, Sherilyn, was a homemaker who always came up with creative or off-the-wall ideas regarding family issues and business ventures. They attended the same church we did.

A few seconds after we all sat down with our lunch trays, Sherilyn got right to the point. "Last night I had a dream about Sherrie and you," she said. "The dream showed me how awful it must be for her to be sick while you have two little kids." So far the conversation was within my comfort zone.

"Then, in the dream, God revealed a plan to me on how to help you guys," she said pushing back her red hair that reminded me of a stop sign. I wished she would stop right there. But the generals and Sherilyns of the world don't stop until they accomplish their missions. Sherilyn's orders, apparently, came from the ultimate Commander-in-Chief.

"Here is what we are going to do to help your family make it through these difficult times," she said. When she said "help" I saw visions of Gary Cooper in "High Noon" and John Wayne in "Stagecoach." Those dudes did not need help. Being raised in the American West myself, I felt that same independent spirit. Sherilyn went on, but my spirit felt as defensive as a middle linebacker during a goal-line stand.

"I woke up in the middle of the night and sat down with paper and pencil while God gave me this plan," she said. I looked around nervously, hoping none of the analytical professionals around us could hear this strange conversation. Steve simply listened with a smile on his face. He knew his wife had shifted into high gear and nothing could stop her. Sherilyn continued.

"We'll work through the church. Helping the Piburns will be the pilot program." Oh, we're the guinea pigs, eh? I thought. This is getting more bizarre by the minute. "I'll have one group made up of families that will each provide one meal per month for your clan, Gregg. I hope to get 16 families to sign up for this part of the program so that you'll have three or four suppers per week. I will also ask them to make a little extra so you can have leftovers the other nights. I will recruit a group of women who will take turns coming in pairs to do house-cleaning once weekly. Finally, I'll line up a group of women and teenagers willing to babysit. All you will have to do is call one number and we'll have a babysitter at your house within an hour."

Her excited face was now as red as her hair. My face was as alive as Abe's on Mt. Rushmore. In the 1970s, I bought Sherrie running shoes and cross-country skis. In the 1980s, I bought her a recliner chair and cordless phone. In the '70s, she won races. In the '80s, she slept 12 hours per day. Sherrie was trying to keep up with two toddlers while having the energy of a weary grandmother. So, God knows we needed the help; I was just too proud and too much of a "caretaker" to admit that to Sherilyn.

"Well, that sounds interesting, Sherilyn, but we don't really need any help," I said. I should have been on horseback while saying those words, pushing up the brim of my hat while flashing a patronizing smile at the schoolmarm who thought she could help the gunslinger. But, the "Colin Powells" of the world don't cave in at the first sign of resistance. "But Gregg, just think how hard it must be for Sherrie," she said, leaning forward to look me square in the eyes. "I really worry about the two of you. I doubt if either of you has the energy to focus on your relationship. This will give you a chance to go on dates, play with your kids, relax a bit while Sherrie gets through the illness. We can continue the program as long as it takes."

"No." My patronizing grin had vanished into the sunset. "Maybe you can try it on a different family." Sherilyn's face remained illuminated by her excitement. "Oh, we'll help many families eventually. But right now your family is the one that needs help."

Many of the employees surrounding our table had completed assertive-management training. But none of them could match Sherilyn when it came to assertiveness. She was the Mike Wallace of the Christian Women's League.

"Listen," I said. "I do appreciate your concern and your willingness to help. But we'll make it just fine. I'm sure there are other families who aren't as well off as we are, who really need it more than we do."

"OK, here's the deal," Sherilyn said. "All I need from you today is a commitment that you will tell Sherrie about the plan and get her thoughts. You don't have to say 'yes' to the program right now." How do you say no to a red-haired fireball that combines the qualities of Colin Powell and Mike Wallace? I took a big breath, then said: "OK, I'll ask Sherrie. But I really doubt that we'll let you do it."

Sherilyn flashed a knowing smile at me. "That's fine; just talk to Sherrie." That night I kept my promise. I told Sherrie about the conversation with Sherilyn. I got the facts right but editorialized plenty through my nonverbals and voice inflection. I assumed that when I finished the explanation we would chat about it for a few minutes before deciding we wanted no part of such a wild program. We would agree that we had no desire to become upper-middle-class beggars.

"So what should I tell Sherilyn?" I asked Sherrie.

"Call her right now and tell her we'll do it," she said. "This is a godsend. We aren't going to survive without help." I swallowed my pride and called.

People in the pseudo-community and chaos phases never think to display a white flag, which they consider a sign of weakness. Sherrie knew we were in need of moving to another level. The level of emptiness. She knew of our unconscious need to call for a surrender, to demonstrate the courage and strength to be vulnerable. Within a week we had our first meal delivered. Two weeks after my call the first housecleaning crew arrived. We rejoiced when our first babysitter arrived, allowing us to go on a long-overdue date. Sherilyn's program served our needs for two years. It went on to help many other church families going through similar trials, too. We knew some of the people on Sherilyn's team, while others were strangers at first. The program conserved our energy, made our difficult lives more bearable, and possibly, just possibly, saved our sanity and our marriage.

We were fortunate to have access to such a support network. Many Americans face their struggles alone. But if there is any way to tap into formal or informal assistance, do so. Let your relationship take precedence over pride. Those western heroes are fictitious. Screenwriters never have their heroes face the realities of illnesses that go on month after month, year after year. I rarely see Sherilyn anymore. But as long as I live I will know she played an angelic role in a wintry season of my life. Tap into an "angel," if one appears.

Medical Maze:
The Needle

— *or* —

Choosing Pain to Ease Pain

L ife was better for Sherrie and the family in late 1996 than it had been for a long time. I picked up a fair dose of superstition while playing 15 years of organized baseball, so I didn't tell people how well Sherrie felt. I hesitated to even dwell on it much in my mind. But the truth was, Sherrie was close to living a normal life for a woman in her early 40s. No, she wasn't going to backpack across the Continental Divide or do back handsprings at the local park. However, she did feel good enough to be in a community play, taking on seven roles while also performing several songs on an accordion. (You had no idea how versatile my wife is, did you?) I sat through the first weekend's performance and marveled at how healthy Sherrie looked. She had some of that old spark back, and joked and laughed with the other cast members after each performance. I could not help thinking that we had finally conquered the worst stretch of the journey. Perhaps, we would soon leave all signs of chronic illness in the dust.

"I'll be consulting at a company in Fort Collins all day," I told Sherrie the morning of Dec. 12, 1996. She replied, "I've got a voice lesson in the morning and I'll rest up all afternoon."

How symbolic for her to be heading to voice lessons. It proved she had overcome so many struggles and could focus her energy now on more positive activities, such as singing, rather than worrying about some future operation. At about 11 a.m. I checked my business voice mail. I heard a friend's voice. "Hi, Gregg, this is Laura. Sherrie is OK, but she got in a car accident this morning between Loveland and Longmont. She called me to pick her up at the hospital. We should be at your house around 12:30 p.m. Don't worry. Bye." I worried . . . big time.

Chronic illness had already taught me that life is difficult. The car accident reminded me that life can become even more trying. I got home before Laura and Sherrie. Every time a car passed our house I ran to the front window to see if it was them. I tried to visualize Sherrie hopping out of the car with a wide grin on her face, exclaiming that she felt fine, not a scratch on her. Being an adept daydreamer, I painted such a realistic picture of that happy scene that I fully expected it to become reality any minute.

A few minutes later Laura's car rolled into our driveway. I came out the front door just as Laura opened Sherrie's door for her. Yes, Sherrie had a smile on her face when she slowly stood up, but it was the plastic grin of a mortuary owner greeting funeral attendees. Sherrie's face tried unsuccessfully to ease my concern. But any hope that the accident was insignificant vanished the second she started to walk toward me. Holding Laura's arm, she took small steps looking like a great-grandmother walking down a bumpy stone path.

Sherrie had stopped at a rural T-intersection. A semi-truck tried to turn in front of her immobile mini-van, but clipped the front end of our vehicle. The truck lifted the van up and dropped it back down. The van bounced up and down and back and forth before coming to a standstill again. Sherrie had already had three spine surgeries and knew something didn't feel right immediately after the van came to a standstill. An ambulance took her to a hospital 10 miles away. X-rays taken there and later on at our doctor's office proved inconclusive. One thing Sherrie knew for sure was that her hips and lower back hurt.

Somehow Sherrie managed to complete her community-theater commitment over the next two weekends. Maybe I was the only person to detect that some of the spark had vanished from her performances. The guitarist had to lift the accordion up to Sherrie's shoulders each time she needed to play and Sherrie had to rest most of each day before rehearsals and performances. Once the play closed, my wife focused her efforts on seeking medical answers to her questions about the discomfort in her hips.

Unfortunately, the answers were far from clear. In early 1997 her orthopedic surgeon, who had performed a neck fusion on Sherrie earlier in the year, said he might have to perform hip surgery but wanted to try other options first. For a few weeks the former long-distance runner used a cane at home and a motorized cart at the grocery store. Sherrie finally told the surgeon she was ready to have him cut her open. "I'm still not convinced surgery is the right step," the surgeon said. "Let's try something else first."

A week or so later Sherrie and I sat in a small room at the local hospital waiting for the surgeon to arrive with a big needle full of a steroid solution. Such injections can relieve pain in sore spots, eliminating the need for surgery.

As I sat beside my wife, I recalled that she had had a steroid injection a few years before for back problems. I remembered that she had gained some relief from the pain in the weeks following that first injection. But I also remembered that Sherrie felt lots of pain during and right after that first injection. I wondered if I would have the guts to purposely choose imminent pain in the hopes of possible relief down the road.

When the doctor arrived and I saw the needle, I felt certain I would have passed on the imminent-pain option. "Uh, wait a second, doc," I imagined myself saying, "I believe I've had a miraculous healing in the past few minutes. Why, I feel little if any pain. There's no need to poke that sharp thing into my healed body."

Alas, Sherrie proved more courageous and wise than I would have been in her situation. She chose to attack her long-term pain by enlisting short-term pain. As the surgeon pressed the needle into Sherrie, I saw her wince. I held her hand and whispered encouragement into her ear. I felt great admiration for this woman who has faced significant challenges for many years of her life. I admired her willingness to face physical and other problems head on.

Pain, of course, isn't confined only to the physical realm. After introducing a group of 20 corporate employees to the four phases, a person asked if there was a simple formula for moving above the barbed wire. "No," I said, "if it was easy, we would all be operating in phases three and four."

People who populate the pseudo-community phase often try to avoid pain or discomfort at any given moment. That avoidance of facing problems head on usually makes the issues more painful and intense. On the other hand, people in the chaos phase might approach the painful spots of life, but often with a win-lose mind-set or a bull-in-the-china-shop demeanor. That chaotic journey to pain sometimes harms other people and relationships.

People who venture into the emptiness of phase three will-fully go directly to the pain. They have the courage to face dis-comfort (or pain) and courageously talk about significant issues others choose to sweep under the rug. They do not toy around with the painful issues of life. They jump right into the middle of each issue, into the middle of the pain. If emptiness has been foreign until then, the pain of going right to the heart of the problem is acute. But it does not usually result in the screams of chaos but in the silence of emptiness. In the midst of phase-three quietness often comes wisdom and healing.

Once you have delved into emptiness, you'll find it easier to go back to it repeatedly. Just as Sherrie's body learned to welcome the pain of the needle – which did relieve some of her pain and, perhaps, helped fight off the need for surgery – you'll begin to welcome the vulnerability and pain of empti-ness, because you know it leads to relational and personal growth.

Life is difficult, full of pain and sorrow. But many people refuse to jump into the center of their discomfort. In the process, they lose out on establishing deeper relationships and the possibility of truly moving beyond their pain.

Parenting:
Delving Into the Nightmare

— *or* —

Hooking a Real Pumpkin

Corlet slept with her 6-year-old face constricted with concern. Behind her closed eyes she saw a kindergarten scene
played out in the strange clarity of a dream. It involved fishing for pumpkins. If you didn't hook a pumpkin, you didn't
get to have a mother.

Three months earlier, in late 1986, Sherrie had her first major
surgery, an oopherectomy. Now, at the age of 33, she was on
the brink of undergoing a second surgery, a hysterectomy.
The gynecologic problems combined with fibromyalgia created a huge dose of anxiety throughout our family of four back
then (we adopted our third child, Bret, nearly two years later).
A certain amount of worry was natural under the circumstances. Fourteen months earlier we had been a family of
healthy individuals. But Sherrie's health problems threw us all
for a loop. It put a strain on our marriage, which is one of
those situations that children mysteriously pick up on, despite
being unable to put it into words.

We had chosen not to tell our young daughters much about
the surgeries. "Mommy is going to go to the hospital so she can
get better," I told them. We didn't feel it necessary to describe

the details of Sherrie's symptoms or what it meant to have surgery – which I believed would have been nearly impossible to describe in terms they could understand anyway. Unfortunately, we also decided to stifle our emotions when talking to our daughters about the operations. We chose this route despite knowing that children can understand feelings such as fear, anger and sadness without our acknowledging them.

Being quite open herself, Sherrie told me about being terrified of undergoing another surgery so soon after her first, which had not remedied her condition. She admitted that she felt extreme loss at not being able to conceive more children. "I've lost so many things already and now I'm losing that option, too. I'm becoming less of a woman," she said. "I know I need the surgery, but I'm angry and sad that I do." Since I was the standard-model "caretaker" back then, I said comforting things such as, "There, there, everything will be all right." I would pat her on the back while I stifled my emotions. However, I'm not sure I knew what my true emotions were, because I focused my energy on fulfilling my "caretaker" role so well. If my mind recognized fleeting emotion, I would quickly bury it with thoughts about what I needed to do next to keep all our lives on an even keel.

One morning I had already left early for work. I had an impressive sounding title, but I'm sure my words and actions on the job that day played no role in making the world a better or worse place. My eight hours of work were insignificant and forgettable. However, Sherrie and Corlet were about to change their worlds.

Corlet awakened with a sick feeling, remembering images of a dream she had just had, which involved a bizarre carnival atmosphere in her classroom. Her classmates took turns throwing a fishing line over a curtain. One by one they reeled in a pumpkin, which meant they got to have a mother. Finally, it was Corlet's turn to hook a pumpkin, except she didn't. When she reeled in her line and jerked it over the curtain, she discovered she had hooked nothing but air. No pumpkin, no mom. Those were the rules of this game.

Lying in bed, feeling that realistic and immense emotion of loss, she started to cry. She got out of bed and ran down the hallway to our bedroom. Sherrie awakened immediately and opened her arms as Corlet leapt into bed and buried her face in Sherrie's chest. Before even asking the reason for the tears, Sherrie began to sob, huge tears fell on the thick, blonde, matted hair of her oldest child.

Like a cloudburst that's rained itself out, mother and child eventually stopped crying. They continued to hold each other as Sherrie said, "What's wrong, Corlet?" Between gasps, Corlet recounted the dream for Sherrie. Then she said: "Mommy, I'm scared about the operation. Will you die?"

Had I been there you know what I would have said. Reading from the "caretaker's" script, I would have replied, "There, there, don't be silly. This is a routine surgery that will make Mommy all better. How about I get you a big bowl of Fruity Pebbles?" Thank goodness I was going through mundane motions in the corporate world.

"No, Corlet, I don't think I will die but I do know I'm scared," Sherrie said.

"Why are you scared?"

Sherrie knew she had a choice to make based on Corlet's question. She could ignore it, lie about it, or respond truthfully to it.

In general, we try to let our kids be kids, not burdening them with adult issues. Sometimes, however, we use this philosophy as an excuse to keep children in the dark. Sherrie chose this day to illuminate our daughter about her operation and her own fears. I'm glad she did.

"I'm scared because they have to cut me with a knife and take out part of my insides. I'm scared because I'll never be able to have more children. I'm scared because I don't want you and Alyse to ever be as sick as I am. I'm scared because the life I thought I would live isn't happening the way I thought it would."

"Tell me more about the operation" Corlet said.

In as basic and accurate a way as possible, Sherrie explained what doctors would do to her in a few days. She also told Corlet what to expect when she got home from the hospital. "I might not ever be as well as I was when you were a baby and pre-schooler," Sherrie said, "but I'll always love you and I will try my hardest to always be here when you need me."

"I'm still kind of scared," Corlet said.

"That's OK, Corlet, because I am, too. We can be scared together."

Later in the day, when Sherrie recalled the conversation, she told me Corlet's tense body softened at her last words – "we can be scared together." She told me they held each other a few more minutes after that and then started talking about kindergarten and friends and little sisters. I'm not positive it started that morning in our bed, but Corlet seems to have always been willing to tell us about whatever is on her mind, to talk from the heart, be it about joy, fear or sorrow. She seems to have learned at an early age that feelings are neither right nor wrong, they just are.

"Thanks, Mommy, I don't feel so scared now."

"I don't either, Corlet."

Intimacy:
Love-Letter Springboards

— or —

Intertwined Hearts & Bodies

In the late 1970s, about six or seven years into our marriage, Sherrie and I attended a Marriage Encounter Weekend, a Christian-based program that helps couples learn how to, among other things, communicate from the heart. One of the tools the instructors of the program used to help couples talk at a deeper level was love letters. The approach involved having husbands and wives write letters to each other in response to specific questions, such as: "How do I feel about the day we first met?" or "How do I feel about you dying someday?" Once the individuals write a letter, they read each other's thoughts. Then they spend time discussing what they wrote and read. It can be a powerful experience.

Unfortunately, Sherrie and I stopped doing the exercise, partially because our lives seemed so easy back then. Years later, however, there came a time when I suggested we use the Marriage Encounter tool to help us deal with an important topic. I knew our sex life had reached a critical point, which forced me to take the initiative to have us write and share love letters. On July 20, 1992, we wrote and read letters in response to the question: "How do I feel about our sex life?"

I boldfaced excerpts from Sherrie's letter and italicized excerpts from mine.

"I feel inadequate, as if I know I've made a commitment to something and then I don't follow through."

"Our sex life disappoints me right now because it seems to take low priority when it comes to what we do on a weekly basis. When we actually do it, I think it is great for both of us, but the task of getting it started seems as difficult as cracking open a textbook on a beautiful Sunday afternoon. It is the tough task of starting that so often prevents the thrill of the journey.

"Many times we have said to each other at the end of love-making, 'We need to do this more often.' In addition, you have told me plenty of times you like it when I take the initiative. At least two reasons I don't take that leap more often come to mind. First, there are so many days and nights you feel exhausted or battle some kind of pain. When you don't feel good, I usually don't feel like making love. I can't get that thought out of my head. Second, by not initiating the activity, I don't have to worry about being turned down. When you say 'no' it hurts my somewhat fragile psyche and cools off my somewhat warmish innards."

"I feel sad. It is like when I do something because I get busy. I'm spinning and twirling and speeding. I don't bother to slow down, to let go, to yield and surrender to the joy and pleasure from God and from you."

"While writing, I realized there might be a solution to the reasons I gave above for not being more of an initiator. If the initiation consists only of a few seconds in the evening as I crawl into bed then I am playing against a stacked deck. A better solution is to be more romantic with you on an ongoing basis, to

show my love for you consistently so that your whole body, mind and spirit will be more attuned to me and the possibilities to come. Just a thought."

"I love you. Sherrie."

"I love you and I love to be next to you and in you. Your lips are so full and soft, and your kisses (to borrow a phrase from King Solomon) are like 'the best wine that goes down smoothly, gliding over lips and teeth.' Humma humma. Gregg."

Sherrie's letter seemed brief and lacked the clarity of her normal writing. The letter seemed a perfect symbol of the exhaustion and confusion she felt at that time in her life. My letter, of course, was far from perfect. But some important words came through in this writing exercise. Words such as inadequate, disappointed, sad, surrender, fragile psyche and fear. Those words and emotions remain buried if a couple gets mired in the pseudo-community phase.

We read the letters and then we talked . . . for a long time. The letters – which in and of themselves seemed quite honest – served as springboards to even greater expressions of truthful communication. Even though we had been married nearly 19 years, we still found it difficult to delve into discussions about sex. The letters, fueled by our emotions, enabled us to talk more openly than ever before about our fears, frustrations and joys surrounding our sex life together.

It took courage, symbolized mainly by our willingness to be vulnerable and delve deeply into the topic, but the more we talked, the easier it became. We came to some specific agreements that day on how we could communicate more openly about sex on an ongoing basis. Explaining those agreements here is unimportant. What is important is that you have this kind of discussion with your significant other, especially if chronic illness has had a negative influence on your sexual relationship.

Something even more powerful happened that day, however. Sherrie and I felt great intimacy toward one another even though we didn't "go all the way." And that warm feeling did not come from the sexual language we spoke. The intimacy came from talking from our hearts, sharing our truths with each other, from deep within our souls.

On Valentine's Day 1998 Sherrie wrote me another letter. She wrote: "It is hard to find the words to express how I feel about you. If you could open me up or see inside, you might see my love for you pouring out. There is not enough room to contain the gladness and joy in my soul.

"I so much appreciate the many hard hours of work you put in every day. Not just for finances, but for parenting partnership. I appreciate the affection, respect and compassion you put so faithfully into our relationship. I am more attracted to you today than in the past. You are the world's greatest lover. I am happy to be the recipient of your loyalty, love and romance. I love you, Sherrie."

Living above "the barbed wire" definitely has (ahem) major advantages. A long time ago, before Sherrie got sick, someone told us lovemaking is a thermometer rather than a thermostat in a relationship. In retrospect, 13 years into Sherrie's health problems, I partially disagree with the statement. Maybe under the circumstances of a normal relationship, it is true. But when something like chronic illness rolls around, I believe loving intimacy can be a way to kick a strained relationship into high gear, just as a thermostat can raise the temperature in a home. Physical intimacy combined with emotional intimacy is a powerful union that can help combat the doubts and losses brought on by chronic illness.

Spiritual:

Seeing with New Eyes

— *or* —

Tapping Into "Sister Death"

Whenever I hop on my motorcycle for a short ride through the nearby prairie or mountains, I take a second to glance behind my left shoulder to see "Sister Death." St. Francis of Assisi called death "sister," a term of endearment for a phenomenon deemed terrible and unspeakable in American culture. By denying the existence of death we limit our options for life. Author and Episcopalian priest Alan Jones writes: "Death, far from being the terror we encounter at the end of our earthly existence, is the companion and friend who walks with us now. Sister Death is with us always. Her shadow marks and influences every moment."

While writing this essay, I looked over my shoulder and again saw "Sister Death." She reminds me that this could be my last day on earth, the last chance I have to write a sentence, to feel the sun on my face, to wrestle with my son, to give a daughter a good-night kiss, to tell Sherrie I love her. "Sister Death" is not so much a token of finality, but rather a symbol that encourages me to improve my quality of life at this moment. While reminding me of my final destination on earth, she helps me appreciate and create a richer journey along the way.

In early 1997 I began to focus more time and energy on the writing of this book. I rediscovered old memories and past lessons related to chronic illness. I plunged into the four phases and again recalled the numbness of living in pseudo-community, the sting of chaos, the relief of emptiness and the power of community. I also tried to practice what I preached in the book. While in the process of writing about becoming more open, honest and courageous with Sherrie, I prodded myself to ask her out on a date. One crisp winter night I took Sherrie to a local establishment, the Summit Restaurant. We sat at a quiet corner table, the softly dim room illuminated by candlelight.

Even though we left the kids at home, I felt the presence of a third person at our table. My beloved Sherrie sat directly across from me. And yet, I saw to my left, out of the corner of my eye, another person – my beloved "Sister Death." She did not have an evil countenance at all. Instead, she looked at me lovingly, then in a subtle move of her head suggested I talk about something important with my wife. While Sherrie looked at the menu, I tried to think about what I wanted to say. I remembered driving down North St. Vrain Canyon in the early stages of our marriage, before children or health problems. "What would you do if I died?" I had asked Sherrie in that younger life we shared. She said she would remain in our house for at least a year. She believed it would take at least that long to work through my death before setting a new course for the rest of her life.

"If you died," I said in my cocksure twenty-something way, "I would quit my job, sell the house and travel the country and the world. That would be how I would deal with your death." What I did not say, but believed, is that I would be able to work through my young wife's death through constant changes of scenery, being exposed to totally new people and processes before finally finding my next comfortable niche. You see, I felt self-actualized back then, seemingly confident that I could find peace and happiness in spite of the circumstances and surroundings. I didn't need the approval of others or the perfection of my environment to gain satisfaction. All I really needed was myself, or so I thought.

Now, as a forty-something year old who had traveled a few bumpy roads in the previous two decades, I had a much different view of life . . . and death. Sherrie and I both possessed accurate memories of the past. I wondered if she still recalled my foolish words about death before I had a clue about life. The waiter took our order and went to get our salads. In the old days, the time between the order and the arrival of the food presented a time for me to show off my charm and humor. My wit had intrigued a few dinner dates during my life. This night, with my wife of 24 years, was not the time to be witty, however. Sister Death suggested a different level of communication.

"Sherrie," I said with the gentleness of a priest about to give last rites, "I want to say something important to you tonight." Her eyes locked on mine with calm anticipation. "Sister Death" leaned forward, putting her elbows on the table. "There have been times in the last 13 years when I felt you would die young," I said. "That feeling has passed, although I know this could be the last day on earth for either one of us." Sherrie nodded her head and conveyed in that simple gesture a longing for me to continue, to quickly delve deeper into the language of the heart.

"My view of life and death has changed much in the last few years. I also have a different view than in my 20s of how I would handle your death," I said. "I want you to know that, because I love you more than I ever thought possible, your death would rip my insides more painfully than I ever imagined. Without you, I'm lost. It might take years to get to the point where I could function again."

Sherrie could have stopped me at any point, interjecting hollow words of comfort. "Oh, I'm not going to die," or "I'm sure you would find a new sweetie within the first month." She chose instead to stay above "the barbed wire" and said nothing.

A 1970s mental picture of me driving away from her funeral in a VW van flashed in my mind for a second. I realized the stupidity of thinking I would blithely drive down the blue highways of America, overcoming my grief as steadily as the movement of the odometer. Alan Jones writes, "When I say to myself, 'This moment may be my last,' I am able to see the world with new eyes."

"Sherrie, I don't want you to think that I'm saying I desperately need you," I said, my voice rising slightly despite the fact others now sat at nearby tables. "I am saying that I want you so much in my life that I can't imagine myself without you." Sherrie continued to gaze into my eyes while her mouth stayed closed.

"I just wanted to tell you those things." Tears now formed in her eyes. "I can clarify what I said if you need me to." A nearly imperceptible shake of her head indicated that would be unnecessary as her eyes continued to lock on mine.

chapter 9

BUSTING
THROUGH THE
DARKNESS

Embracing problems goes against the nature of many people, including me. But if you break through that barrier, powerful things can happen to you and to your relationships.

Tick, Tock, Sob, Tock

— or —

The Midnight Hug

My eyes flew open, but all I saw was the panther-black blanket of night that covered our bedroom. I felt disoriented as I tried to understand why I had awoken. My mind was scrambled like a firefighter aroused from sleep by a siren in the dead of night. But my body was frozen with fear, as if I were trapped in a nightmare being chased by lumbering cadavers. My mind knew something was amiss, while my body awaited instructions. All I heard was tick, tock, tick, tock from the clock nearby.

How can a man sitting in the upper deck spot an offensive lineman moving an instant before the center snaps the ball, but not detect that his wife has dropped into the funk of depression? How can a person take corporate-sponsored sensitivity training but be blind to the fact a loved one lives in fear of some nameless, faceless enemy? How can people get so concerned about the gnats buzzing around their heads that they often ignore the elephants bearing down on their significant others?

My heart seemed to stop and my ears felt as if they had been stretched toward the ceiling in an attempt to decipher what I thought I heard in my sleep. I held my breath, trying desperately to catch some movement or sound that would give me a clue about what was wrong. Tick, tock, tick, tock, sob, tock. There it was, 10 inches away from my head. Sherrie had stifled a cry in the night. Then I felt her whole body shake with the subtlety of an aspen leaf blown by a slight breeze. For 30 more seconds I listened to Sherrie's internal struggle, partially out of curiosity and partially because I didn't know how to help.

Man's instinct is to solve the problem. The emotionless executive inside me wanted to bolt out of bed, flick on the light, set up a bedside flip chart, ascertain the situation and gain consensus for a four-step action plan designed to solve the problem. "There, that's settled. Now let's see if we can get a little more shut-eye before sunup." Marshall Matt Dillon as facilitator. The Gen. George Patton School of Counseling. A proud graduate of the Hulk Hogan Sensitivity Workshop.

Maybe because my mind couldn't click to attention and march to its routine of masculine orders at that late hour of the night, I kept the light off and my mouth shut. After a while though I rolled over and faced my wife, silently wrapping my arms around her like a child hugging a favorite teddy bear.

In this era of The Rational Man and Woman, when the mind rules, we often forget the power of simple, nonsexual touch. Mother Teresa once said, "We can do no great things; only small things with great love."

When I made Sherrie my teddy bear, her muffled weeping turned into thunderous sobs combined with torrential tears. I continued to squeeze her, saying nothing. After 30 seconds the downpour of tears turned into steady rain, then sprinkles, then the calm after the storm, then sleep. Throughout the whole time, our lips and bodies remained still.

I am a full-time communication professional, making speeches and writing essays for a living. My mouth sprints at the microphone and my fingers fly on the keyboard. But my greatest communication achievement occurred on a still, dark night when no words slipped through my lips. In the years that have passed since that night, I never asked Sherrie why she was crying and she never felt the need to tell me.

Just before her steady, slow breathing tugged me back to sleep, I gave her one more gentle squeeze. We would make it through the night and face tomorrow.

The Critics' Choice

— or —

80 mph & Climbing

One allure of playing the "caretaker" role is that it often draws rave reviews. Occasionally a person would say something such as: "Gregg, how do you do it? You have so much responsibility, but you seem so calm, so in control. I'm very impressed."

I drew the equivalent of standing ovations from those around me. No wonder it seemed so natural and rewarding to play this starring role. In some cases, an actor's stage role replaces the person's real identity in the public's mind. To many people, Yul Brynner is The King and Hal Holbrook is Mark Twain and Candace Bergen is Murphy Brown. Back in the late '80s, Gregg Piburn was the "Caretaker." I sensed people around me saw and appreciated Gregg Piburn in that role. In the process, I began to lose my identity, to the point that my "caretaker" role took precedence over the real person.

Even though Yul, Hal and Candace are masters of their craft, they still read occasional nasty reviews by critics. It's easy to ignore the critics, but many great actors ponder reviews to discover hidden nuggets. Within my throng of admirers, I also had a few critics.

Sherrie: "When are you going to really open up and be honest with me?"

Corlet: "Why do you always have to act like you're perfect?"
Alyse: "Why are you gone so much of the time?"
Bret: "Why can't you play with me? It's Saturday."
I also had another critic, my buddy and co-worker John. He was not afraid to pan my "caretaker" performance and push my envelope. John and I often took drives in the company car to talk a little business and a lot of life. One gray day, John and I were driving on a two-lane road through the Colorado prairie. We were returning from a speaking engagement and our conversation turned to personal issues. (This conversation was so important to my journey that I include it in the Introduction and here.)

"Gregg, how does it make you feel to have Sherrie sick for so long?" John asked. Unlike other friends and acquaintances, John was not afraid to dig deep into my psyche, which felt abused by my wife's chronic conditions.

"Well, I certainly feel sad, especially for Sherrie," I answered. "But, you know, I'm sad for the kids and me, too." The car's speedometer read 60 mph.

"You're thinking too much," John said, jabbing my shoulder with his fist, which was the size of a linebacker's. "What does your heart say?" I began to understand how people feel when Mike Wallace interviews them. "OK," I said, "I'm mad – mainly at the conditions." 65 mph.

"What about her operations?" I squeezed the steering wheel and remained silent. "C'mon," John pleaded, "don't clam up on me now!" Bingo!

"Yeah, I've got feelings," I screamed. "Like when I think of hospitals, I get scared. After every one of the operations

Sherrie looks dead or close to dying. Her lips are white, her hair is matted and her speech is slurred. She wears her pain on her face. White-smocked doctors walking around like they were gods, cutting open my wife and sewing her back up, making the obligatory summary speech to me in the waiting room, always saying things went great, acting as if they had swooped down from heaven to save the damn day." 75 mph.

"At least Sherrie slept through much of that crap. I'm the good little boy who had to sit in those putrid waiting rooms with my little laptop computer so I could write how wonderful it would be when the royal doctors would get done and everything would be like the old days. Pecka pecka pecka peck peck."

John said, "Now we're getting somewhere. What has it really been like?"

"For years nobody asked me that question! Everybody wants to know how Sherrie is, but what about me? We were always going to be so independent. For months we had people bringing meals, sending cards, watching the kids, scrubbing toilets. I thanked them for doing it, but hated them having to. Then they wanted to give me money. I didn't need their damn money! I needed Sherrie to get well and I needed to let my own guard down – instead of always acting so cool, so in control, so strong. I . . . am . . . just . . . plain . . . pissed!"

We topped out at 90 mph and silence filled the car. Then I took a deep breath – the breath of a prisoner set free.

It took a while to rid myself of the "caretaker" role. But during that law-breaking drive on the prairie my closest friend and critic helped me begin to wash off the phony make-up and shred the unhealthy mind-set that I donned when Sherrie got sick. In the following days I decided to explore a different character, the real me, set free from the bonds of a script. Living without a script gave me more opportunities for personal growth and, ironically, helped me be a better support person for Sherrie. If life is the ultimate story, I would rather write my own scenes than follow a preconceived plot written by someone else. Set yourself free.

A Learning Philosophy

— *or* —

A Teflon Shield

I stood in front of 175 business people from New Hampshire one spring day in 1995. A national training company
had solicited my consulting services to do workshops for various audiences around the country. I always feel extremely
comfortable and confident presenting my own material, but
never feel at ease leading sessions developed by others. I also
dreaded giving a sales pitch for motivational tapes and videos
I had been asked to promote. Leading up to my debut as a
tape pitch man, I gave a brief lecture on ethics, describing
differences between I-it and I-you relationships. In the former, I treat you well only if I think there is something in it
for me. You become merely an object to help me get something I want (money, a job or sex, for example). In the I-you
relationship, we treat each other with honesty and respect because, as human beings, we both deserve that kind of treatment.

Just as I finished that section of the workshop, I noticed it
was time to smoothly ease into my brief marketing presentation before the morning break. Three sentences into my pitch,
a woman yelled, "Oh, this is where you start treating us like an
'it.'" She stunned me with her accurate criticism. A second
later, a person seated next to her said, "I am greatly offended
by what you are doing and do not intend to come back after

the break." I felt like a boxer whose legs become rubbery after receiving a strong one-two combination to the head. Despite being an experienced public speaker, trainer and group facilitator, I panicked when I got forced into the ropes.

"Uh, gee I'm sorry you feel that way." I felt 350 eyeballs aimed straight at my red face. "Uh, look, um, don't feel obligated to buy anything. You know, I personally would prefer not having to talk about the tapes, but it's part of my agreement to do so. But really, you only should buy something if you really want it. I, uh, hope you both come back after the break." Sales were not brisk that day. Amazingly, the two critics did come back, although I would not have done so after the shabby way I reacted to the criticism. I felt like that punch drunk boxer who flails weakly with both arms in a desperate attempt to stay alive until the end of the round.

Three days later on the plane trip home I thought about how I could prevent that sorry scene from recurring. Sometime during that four-hour flight I came up with the following statement: "Whatever happens, use it as a learning or teaching opportunity." This one philosophy has boosted my confidence while also helping to boost my consulting business. In a minute, I'll show you how it affects my personal life. Before the plane landed I visualized what the New Hampshire scene would have looked like had I put the philosophy into practice.

"Oh, this is where you start treating us like an 'it.'"

I would have replied: "It took a lot of courage to say that. Now help the group and me understand exactly what it was I did or said that made you feel like an 'it.'"

In my visual drama, I noticed the 350 eyeballs quickly moving from me to the critic. I became "Teflon Facilitator," at least in my fictional vignette. I also imagined how my reply would have been the springboard to a wonderful discussion, a chance to "turn on the lights." Instead of a dry lecture about ethics, we would have created a group discussion about an event we all experienced moments before. Ethics come alive! It seemed valid in my head, but now I needed to test my theory on a real audience.

Fifteen engineers sat in a circle around me. After five minutes of describing my plan for the day's workshop, a large man with a scowling face said, "May I say something before we move on?" I said, "Sure."

"I think everything you have said until now is bullshit." Thirty eyeballs zoomed in on me.

"First," I said in a confident, non-sarcastic voice, "I have to commend you for having the guts to say something like that. As a facilitator, I create an open and honest environment and you just got us off to a fast start. The last thing I want to do today is create a B.S. environment. Now help the group and me understand what it was I did or said that made it seem like bullshit." Thirty eyeballs now refocused on the critic.

He hesitated a few seconds, scrambling to find the right words. Then he explained why he said it. I clarified something he misunderstood from my original comments and we had an excellent conversation about a couple of other points. Then we moved forward to the next section of the session and I sensed everyone realized this was going to be a different kind of retreat.

Back at home, my son was struggling with intense tantrums for reasons we could not pinpoint. For a few months my family of five seemed controlled by a young boy who was only belt high. I felt as if his anger formed a dark cloud over our house and our psyches. I grew angry at the situation and angry at Bret. Nothing good, I told myself, could come from this ongoing storm of punches, screams and curses. At the same time that Bret was upsetting the household with his tantrums, Sherrie was trying to recover from her car accident. We both felt hopeless, so our conversations led us down blind alleys. It took the wisdom of a friend with an outside perspective to help me change my mindset.

I called John one morning because I needed to let off some steam, lots of steam. "I'm going crazy," I told John, a bachelor living in a small Oregon farmhouse. "Bret has this whole family in his grip, holding us tightly by the proverbial balls." John and I rarely hold back when we speak to each other from the head and heart. I went on by giving some examples of Bret's behavior and how it was affecting our family. I did not expect or demand advice from my longtime confidant. I just needed to spew some of the venom that had developed inside me during Bret's recent spells of misbehavior. But John took a chance by being honest with me. "I wonder what Bret and life are trying to teach you, Gregg. I've seen you struggle with other issues, make changes in your life and become a better man for it. God, or fate, or life, whatever you want to call it, finds you an able student willing to learn and grow. So he throws plenty of lessons your way. My advice is that you not view Bret as this tiny troublemaker, but a gift from God who has some powerful things to teach you."

John's words felt like cool salve applied to raw wounds. Even as he spoke, I sensed my view of Bret becoming softer, more loving than it had been in recent weeks. John's words became prophetic because Sherrie and I grew through the process of helping Bret work through his anger. We learned powerful lessons about perseverance, love and peace in the eye of the storm. We also learned about chemical imbalance and medication that helps ease the anger while keeping the mind sharp.

I use my philosophy "Whatever happens, use it as a learning or teaching opportunity," a few times monthly in my work. If I stay true to myself, I can use it daily as a part of my personal life. Chronic illness, of course, offers plenty of chances to put my theory of life to work. Many lessons prove difficult. But I would rather learn and grow from them, than cower and stagnate. My advice to you: "Whatever happens, use it as a learning or teaching opportunity."

Responding to Emotions

— *or* —

How to Handle a Loaded Weapon

You must be careful with a loaded weapon. A handgun, for example, has the potential to be greatly beneficial (saving a loved one from injury or death) or greatly harmful (causing the injury or death of a loved one). Being more attuned to and talking about emotions has the potential for good and bad outcomes as well. Here are two ways to improve the odds that the way you respond to emotions gleans positive results.

1. How to convey emotions with others.

"You torque me off."

"You really screwed up this time."

"You and your illness are making my life a living hell."

What are some of the similarities between the three statements above? Tick, tick, tick. Time's up. Here are two similarities that make the loaded weapon of expressing emotions potentially damaging to relationships.

First, the speaker uses the word "you" in expressing the emotion. And when you hear someone else refer to you in a negative context, you're likely to get defensive. One of the statements above followed by a defensive retort from the other person quickly drives a conversation into the red zone.

"You torque me off."

"Oh yeah, well if you weren't so thin-skinned maybe you wouldn't always fly off the handle."

This dialogue is taking two people on a fast flight to Trouble City. How could you express emotions more effectively? Turn the "you"s into "I"s.

"I feel angry about the way you treated the last customer."

"I feel confused about the way the process changed."

"I feel sad about what chronic illness is doing to us."

Remember, feelings are neither right nor wrong, they just are. You are not a bad person for feeling angry, confused or sad. Historian and TV documentary producer Ken Burns says, "If it has no emotion, it has no meaning." By telling others how you feel, you provide more information to enhance understanding between the listener and you.

In these last three statements the initial focus is on the speaker rather than the listener. This reduces the need to get defensive. Notice the latter three statements leave more room for explanation and meaningful dialogue. The second similarity of the first three statements is the speaker sounds judgmental. He or she leaves no room for the possibility that the listener could be right. For example, on closer inspection we may discover that the listener did not "screw up" at all. People don't like others to judge them and will often respond to the judgment by spitting and cussing. Judging can also be harmful when approached positively.

"I'm pregnant."

"That's wonderful!" you say with a huge grin.

In truth, being pregnant might be extremely bad news for the woman who started the conversation. At this point, however, you have probably blocked any meaningful communication.

You could respond more effectively by asking an open-ended question that opens the gateway to communicating on a higher emotional level. These questions begin with the words who, what, when, where, why or how.

"I'm pregnant."

"How do you feel about that?"

Now you have built a framework for valuable discussion.

When trying to speak with others on an emotional level, use "I" statements rather than "you" statements. In addition, consider using open-ended questions rather than judgmental statements.

2. How to respond internally to your emotions.

First, remember the premise that feelings are neither right nor wrong, they just are. You can't prevent emotions from surfacing. Just try to keep from being sad the next time a beloved pet dies or try to refrain from anger the next time a crazy driver cuts you off. Where you shine or falter is the way in which you respond to your emotions. Second, take responsibility for your emotions. Tune in to your feelings and tell yourself you are responsible for what you do with them.

I am angry because Clint changed the process. Now I tell myself, "I'm responsible for what I do with that anger." Hmm, I could fret or stew about the situation or I could go to Clint and use "I" statements and open-ended questions to create a meaningful discussion. I am sad about Sherrie's illness. Hmm, I could hold it all in until that sadness turns into anger directed at Sherrie, or I could have the courage to tell her how I feel and make our relationship even richer. The next time you recognize a strong feeling inside you, follow up by telling yourself, "I'm responsible for what I do with that emotion." You'll sense more calmness and wisdom within yourself. A counselor told Sherrie and me a few years ago that we had become adept at handling times of crisis. "It's the in-between times that cause you two trouble," he added. By continually speaking openly about your feelings and practicing the four suggestions below, you can make the in-between times opportunities for personal and relational growth.

1. Use "I" statements rather than "You" statements.
2. Ask open-ended questions instead of making judgmental statements.
3. Remember the premise that feelings are neither right nor wrong, they just are.
4. Take personal responsibility for how you respond to your feelings.

A White-Flag Victory

— or —

Breaking the Grief Barrier

Whew! The kids finally succumbed to bedtime and Sherrie and I had a few minutes before we hit the hay ourselves. The spouse's life often mirrors the roller-coaster symptoms of the person with chronic illness. Sherrie felt better so I did, too. Life is good, I thought, as I reveled in the evening's peace. Frankly, I felt like vegetating in front of the tube, but Sherrie suggested a different course of action. A few weeks before we had started doing a communication exercise that had helped us grow closer through the challenges of chronic illness. Two or three nights weekly we took turns talking for 15 minutes each without interrupting each other. We gave each other permission to share any thought or feeling. The listener's job entailed listening, nothing more.

On this night, I started. I talked to Sherrie about how great it felt to see her doing better. I talked about how peaceful and satisfying it is to know our three children were safely asleep in our house. I talked about job frustrations, feeling trapped in a good-paying job that involved only low-level effort. I conveyed no major news flashes. It was a good, though bland, news update of my life. Then it was Sherrie's turn.

She started where I left off. She talked about her day. She admitted to some frustrations about child discipline. She said she also appreciated the peacefulness of knowing our kids were safe. Nothing major here, I thought, as my mind started to drift.

"There's something else I have not wanted to tell you," she said. Uh-oh. I mentally flinched as one familiar with periodic slaps of negative news from Sherrie. "But I need to tell you. I found a lump in my breast and will have it checked tomorrow." These words were not a slap but a vicious, closed-fisted punch to the rib cage. She sat motionless on the couch five feet from my chair. Her eyes caressed mine, but her lips did not move. The only thing I heard was the stillness of the night. The whole earth had joined my children in slumber. But my mind raced. For the last several years, every doctor's prognosis proved overly optimistic. Projected minor pain turned into big-time hurt. Projected outpatient surgeries turned into major surgeries with lengthy hospital stays. Projected short setbacks became long, overcast seasons.

My mind transformed a lump on the breast to a death sentence. The "Big C" – cancer – overwhelmed my thoughts. Sherrie sat as still as a statue while my mind raced. All I could think was Sherrie had cancer and would die young. I had feared this medical marathon would end with "The Big C." Now reality was merging with those fears. For a second I had a strange urge to tell Sherrie about my fear. But old lessons and common sense slapped me across the face. She does not need Dr. Gloom to give her a prognosis now. You don't tell the woman you love you think she is going to die. What I really wanted to tell her was this: "Don't worry, hon, everything will be just fine and dandy. Hey, 'Cheers' is about to begin. Let me switch on the TV."

"The male beast is . . . well, a dumb beast for the most part.
We don't listen, we don't talk, we don't feel, we don't live. We
analyze, we present, we play the angles, we work."
— *Journal excerpt: Jan. 27, 1988.*

More silent seconds ticked by before a small voice whispered inside my head. "Well, if you are dishonest and gutless you won't tell the woman you love you think she's going to die. Don't you ever tire of that walking-on-eggshells brand of existence? It hasn't worked well for 40 years. Are you going to stay with that mode of operation for the next 40?" I crashed through old barriers. I took a deep breath and leaned forward, ready to display my white flag, and stared into Sherrie's teary eyes.

"I'm scared, Sherrie. I'm afraid they'll find cancer and I think you'll die young."

She looked stunned even though the features of her statue-like face barely moved. Oh man, I thought, I blew it.

Then she said: "For the last two days the thought of death has scared me. But there is something even more terrifying to me. It's going through the death process without you emotionally by my side. Now I know you're with me and will always be with me. I'm scared, too, but I know I'm not alone." I listened, I talked, I felt, I lived. A few days later we found out the lump was benign and we celebrated one day of victory.

SECTION THREE ACTION PAGE:
Reflect ... Then Act!

You will notice this action page demands more courage and energy than previous pages. Remember, most organizations, teams, families and individuals just bounce back and forth between the phases of pseudo-community and chaos. Busting through "the barbed wire" takes effort that will pay huge dividends in the game of life.

1. Develop a losses list

In the first chapter of this section, I wrote an essay titled "Dealing with Denial *or* A Losses List." I listed eight major losses Sherrie and I have suffered since "The Intruder" entered our lives. List some of your losses, along with a brief explanation of how those losses have impacted you and what you will do about dealing with them.

2. Begin a journal

Write daily entries for at least two weeks. It is only for your eyes. Neither your seventh-grade English teacher nor I will look for grammatical errors. Consider journal writing as a way of lassoing those rambling, light-speed thoughts and feelings and putting them into an 8 1/2-by-11-inch corral. An entry might be a paragraph or 12 pages in length. Your mind and your heart will decide. Mine are usually about a page long. The journal helps you get started or improves your ability to recognize your feelings about various situations and people in your life. The following questions might serve as prompts to help you start this 14-day trial run.

- How do I feel about starting a journal?
- How do I feel about the most poignant statement I heard someone say today?
- How do I feel about the way I handled a tough situation today?
- How do I feel about the challenges I'll face in the coming week?
- How do I feel about the way my significant other (or friend, or child) and I interacted today?
- How do I feel about my career and its impact on my entire life?
- How do I feel about what chronic illness is doing to my life right now?
- How do I feel about the argument I had yesterday with (whomever)?
- What is my biggest hope for today (or tomorrow)?
- How do I feel about the losses I have suffered due to chronic illness?
- What did I learn from the disappointment of yesterday?
- If I could go anywhere and do anything today, what would I do and why?
- If I were perfectly honest, what do I REALLY feel about chronic illness?
- What gives me the greatest sense of hope about my (or our) future?

By answering these questions (or questions similar to these) you are choosing to discover who you really are. True, that could be terrifying, but imagine what it must be like to get to the end of your life and realize how little you know about yourself. Do some self-exploration during the next 14 days.

3. Talk, then listen ... or ... listen, then talk

Set aside 30 minutes some evening soon so that you and your significant other can talk to each other for 15 minutes respectively, without interruptions. Talk about anything, but I hope you both begin to share some feelings about important issues, such as chronic illness. When one person is talking, it is important that the other person do nothing but listen. Warning: At first it might be tough for the talker to keep talking and it might be hard for the listener to keep quiet. Try to work through that, though, because free uninterrupted speech and focused attention to the speaker is crucial to this activity's success.

4. Write a magical exchange of letters

This, another writing exercise, can be a powerful way to get in touch with your feelings and walk away with a different perspective on a key aspect of your life. Follow the directions below. If possible, do not read ahead. In other words, do not read the next direction until you have done all the previous steps.

A. Picture the face of a person you consider to be a mentor, a sage and/or a loved one. This person can be living or dead.

Whoever it is, you believe the person is wise and cares for you. For example, I pictured my Grandma Stewart who died two days after my college graduation when I first did this activity as part of a journal entry.

B. Now picture that person in a place in which they did or would find comfort – a college classroom, a farmhouse kitchen, in the back of a pick-up truck, a cozy den.

C. On a sheet of paper, write a letter to that person with the understanding that he or she will read it in that comfortable place noted in **B**. I would like you to focus your letter on the impact of chronic illness on your life. Tell that mentor/ sage/loved one your deepest thoughts and feelings about that topic. If appropriate, ask for advice.

D. Take a five-minute break away from your letter.

E. Now, again picture the person you wrote the letter to in his or her comfortable place. Read the letter you just wrote, pretending you are that mentor/sage/loved one in that special place.

F. Take another five-minute break.

G. One more time, I want you to picture the person you wrote the letter to in his or her comfortable place. Now I want you to again pretend you are that mentor/sage/loved one, but this time I want you to write a letter to yourself, a letter of reply to the first one you wrote. Since you have gotten in touch with that person during this exercise, I believe you will have found just the right words to put into the reply letter. The words you write will seem as if they really did come from that mentor/sage/loved one.

H. Take another five-minute break.

I. Read over the reply letter, then write a journal entry explaining your thoughts and feelings about what you learned from the exercise.

J. If your mentor/sage/loved one is dead, be thankful you could still find a way to connect with him or her. If they are alive, consider sending your first letter to him or her. You may choose to edit the letter somewhat before mailing it.

5. Mine for gold

• Out of all the essays and suggested activities in this chapter, which one contains the most significant and/or memorable nugget for you?

_____

_____

_____

• What is the "first step" you will take toward making that nugget truly impact your life for the better?

• I will _____ (what?)

by _____ (when?)

EXAMPLE: I will write a magical exchange of letters (#4 above) by the end of the week.

FIGHTING BACK, IN THE LIGHT

(phase four

Community. Populated by real people. Epitomized by honesty, conflict resolution, relationships.)

"We've got problems, so let's attack them head on."

chapter 10

SEEKING THE
TRUTH

Truth comes in many shapes and forms,
thanks to messengers of many shapes and
forms.

Silent Lies

— or —

Hard Lessons on the Hard Truth

Your idea of love better change over the years or you'll be in big trouble. The puppy love of fourth grade must be different from the dog-eared love of long-term marriage, for example. All I wanted from Lee Ann in elementary school was an occasional smile and a chance to walk her home once a week. All I want from Sherrie is everything about her, forever. Being involved in a long-term relationship is a whole new dimension, involving a whole lot of commitment from both of us. In addition, I've learned to approach honesty in a new way. I used to think distinctions between honesty and dishonesty were as clear as night and day.

My simple definition of lying used to be, "Purposely saying something you know to be untrue." My view of lying expanded after a few tough lessons from Professor Sherrie. Like many people, I tend to clam up when things get tense. The situation is hard enough, why make it more difficult by bringing up thoughts and feelings that might add more tension? Remember, choosing comfort over discomfort at any given moment is a natural human trait, especially for those who reside in the phase of pseudo-community. This reliance on silence seems especially apt if you, as a "caretaker," wish to protect the china doll who is the "patient." Many people blindly follow this terse and repressive script, believing that in the process they are as honest and true blue as an Eagle Scout, as pure and noble as Mother Teresa.

My "china doll" Sherrie, who is anything but that, strongly disagreed with my mum (or perhaps a better word is "cowardly") way of handling tense situations. And she found an exceptionally pointed way to get her honest message across. It took about two or three sessions for the lessons to sink in, but I now understand her thoughts on the matter. Boy do I understand.

A typical session went like this. My wife and I are clearing the dinner dishes and putting leftovers into the refrigerator. She starts asking me open-ended questions such as, "How do you feel about my upcoming surgery?" or "What are you doing to take care of yourself?" My answers reflect my caveman ancestry as they consist of muffled one- or two-word grunts designed to halt this line of questioning and move us to safer topics of conversation, such as the night's TV schedule or her assessment of the latest Denver Broncos victory.

Holding a stack of dirty dishes, I head for the sink, but my wife intercepts me before I get there. With one hand she grabs a handful of shirt collar and chest hair. Through clenched teeth she says: "You are so full of crap. Tell me what you really think and feel about it." With the index finger of her other hand she begins poking my clavicle. She definitely has my attention with this in-your-face instructional philosophy. "At this point," she continues, "I don't even care if you tell me a bunch of B.S." That's not exactly true, because when I try that approach she pinches and pokes even harder. "I want to know that you are still alive by telling me something meaningful," she says.

"Ooowwww," I say at last. Her hand lets go of my chest, but her eyes stay glued to mine. Then I talk and it is not B.S. I tell her how much I hate seeing her in the recovery room looking like a store mannequin. I tell her I haven't even thought about my own physical or mental health for weeks. I tell her how scared or mad or sad or excited or whatever I am. The moment I begin speaking the truth, the hard outer shell of "Professor Sherrie" instantly vanishes and she becomes engrossed in my words. Afterward, she thanks me for being honest, for painting a vivid picture of where I am at that given moment. Keeping the picture from her represents dishonesty in her mind. I have now come over to that way of thinking myself, even though it creates a much higher standard for what it means to be truthful.

You might be thinking you can't have a relationship in which you are totally open all the time. I agree with that statement, but it is a philosophy we erroneously push to the limit, giving ourselves permission to hide many truths instead of bringing them to light. Before the lessons Sherrie taught me, I always leaned toward the side of silence. Now, if I'm to err, I hope it is by saying a bit more than necessary. Dr. William Masters, of Masters & Johnson fame, once described good communication in a relationship as "the privilege of sharing vulnerabilities." Broaden your idea of honesty and you will broaden your relationships.

Beyond Magic & Miracles

— *or* —

The Battle Cry

A giant in the field of corporate training once leaned over to me and said, with a sly grin, "Of course, our industry's little secret is that many nationwide trainers are hypocrites who rarely if ever do what they say." Trainers don't have a monopoly on hypocrisy. There must be nutritionists who pig out behind closed doors, drill sergeants who cry at sentimental McDonald's TV commercials and financial advisers who have never created a personal budget. The list could go on and on, and would certainly include authors.

A similar phenomenon occurs with organizations, work teams and families. A group will go through intensive training about some topic. Many or all group members will get excited about the learning and resolve to implement some of the key teachings into their careers or lives. They'll talk a good game for a few days or weeks, but eventually all signs of the learning vanish.

Every day I have a chance to test whether I really believe what I write in this book. Most of the time I pass the test, but there are times when I slip.

Several months after Sherrie's van was struck by a truck, Sherrie went in for a myelogram. She considered this a precursor to yet another spine surgery. Without even thinking, I went into my old pseudo-community mode of operation – distancing myself from Sherrie, grieving alone, getting busy with tasks. In times of difficulty or crisis, humans usually go into "back-up mode," doing what comes naturally, what we've done thousands of times in the past. We forget recent lessons learned and let unhealthy habits formed long ago rule the difficult days of the present. Fortunately, Sherrie saw what was happening and encouraged me to talk about my feelings.

"You look worried," she said while lying on a hospital bed waiting for the myelogram to begin. I nodded but said nothing, hoping the conversational path Sherrie envisioned would lead to a quick dead end. I felt like a 7-year-old boy whose mother wants to tease and cajole him out of his little pouting spell. Even as his little mouth forms into a smile at the mother's prodding, his brain is shouting, "Get out of my face, let me pout!" I wanted to silently pout about this latest of Sherrie's many physical setbacks, which represented another emotional setback for the family. In all honesty, I felt like a little boy in a 200-pound body who just wanted to be left alone. But Sherrie sought to release my true emotions and raise me up from the level of the pseudo-community phase through to the phases of emptiness and community.

Sherrie didn't let me off the hook. My nod told her I had plenty of anxieties as I sat next to her hospital bed. "Come on, Gregg, please tell me what you are thinking and feeling?" It would have been so easy to say something such as, "No, I'm fine, just tired." It would have taken so little effort to short-cut this conversation. And a big part of me truly wanted to do it. I could easily have chosen comfort over discomfort at that moment, perhaps without even angering Sherrie. But I decided to practice what I preach.

I opened up and told her of my guilt at always being the one beside the hospital bed, rather than the one in it. I told her how disappointed I was about her latest setback, especially after she had been doing so well. I confessed that her latest health problems made it difficult to focus on my consulting business, which made me worry that financial hardship could be around the next bend. During that usually horrible time of waiting, we had a wondrous and far-ranging conversation about our fears . . . and our hopes.

A couple of months after the myelogram, I went with Sherrie to an appointment with her surgeon, who was still trying to determine whether Sherrie needed to have another surgery. I asked tough questions and received straight answers. The surgeon believed it was too early for surgery and suggested other measures to ease or eliminate her pain. That night, Sherrie knew I felt tired and stressed. "Do you want to go for a walk?" she asked. I wanted to stay planted on the couch. However, I also knew Sherrie did not want to go through this next chapter of her illness alone. "Yes, let's go," I said.

On our walk we did not develop some creative action plan for the coming months. We did not whisper Romeo-and-Juliet statements of love in each other's ears. We did not make any important decisions. We talked about many things – some significant, some trivial. We chuckled a few times. We held hands a while. We had periods of silence. And when we got back to our porch we felt loved and calm. We felt united. "We can do this," Sherrie said to me once we got into the house. It was her way of saying we would overcome the challenges of her latest health problems.

Earlier I alluded to the challenge of helping organizations, teams and families remember and implement the key lessons they have learned from various situations in their lives. As a corporate consultant, I often help companies create pithy battle cries that inform, remind and inspire those employees to keep going no matter how hard the tasks assigned them may be. Some recent groups I worked with came up with the following slogans: "Break out of the box," "UnderStand & deliver" and "It's a whole new game" Sherrie and I started using the phrase "We can do this" as our subtle battle cry.

When we are forced to use our slogan, the word "this" sometimes refers to dealing with chronic illness. More accurately, however, "this" represents life. We can do THIS. I like our battle cry because it promotes hope for our future without demanding or expecting magic or miracles. We can DO this. When we unite, Sherrie and I can and will face what life dishes out to us. WE can do this. It will take love and perseverance and commitment and faith and hard work. It won't be easy and we won't always be totally successful, but . . . we CAN do this.

Break Out of the Box

— or —

Messages from Anywhere

In April 1998, Bret and I attended the wedding of a buddy's son. In the middle of the service, the Lutheran minister improvised by having the bride and groom turn away from him and face the 400 guests. "Look out there, Shelley and Ryan, and see the faces of your loved ones who came tonight," the minister said. The couple smiled sheepishly as they looked across the crowded sanctuary.

"You WANTED them here tonight for this auspicious event, but you will NEED them alongside you for the rest of your life, which is the more important 'event.'" The minister's words struck a chord as the faces of the bride and groom grew introspective. "Frankly, without significant help from others, I don't give this or any marriage much chance of survival."

Unfortunately, many couples fear seeking help from other sources because they view it as a sign of weakness. Perhaps they assume their great love for one another will carry the day, help them overcome all of life's difficulties. There might be a few rock-solid, much-blessed couples who can succeed on their own, but the vast majority of the mortal rest of us need to tap into other resources for support.

Sherrie and I sat in the office of our counselor. That's right, our "shrink." It seems odd that society throws such a belittling and confining term onto the counseling profession, but they do. I associate the word "shrink" with being stuffed into a box. I find that good counselors help you bust out of the restrictive boxes many couples create from their own fear, ignorance, hopelessness and old ways of thinking. When I sometimes hesitated to break out of the box of pseudo-community, Roy, our counselor, possessed the assertive skill to get me to open up. At the end of one particular session he told me, "I believe you want people to say how much they appreciate your efforts and accomplishments," he said. "I'm not saying it is wrong for you to want that." I knew Roy and Sherrie saw me swallow the emotion that would have brought my tears to the session.

The tears came a few minutes later as I drove home. "You are God's greatest gift to me," Sherrie said. "I appreciate you as a husband and as a wage earner." Sherrie's gentle words made me want to turn on windshield wipers for my eyelids. I then started to praise Sherrie for her love and toughness, but she stopped me. "Just listen for a while." I wiped my eyes with the sleeve of my jacket. "The kids love you, but they don't love your career. They still need you to tuck them in at night, to take them on special outings, one-on-one. We all want you, the real you, more than anything else."

I drove on in silence for a half-mile before saying, "Did you just give me some more to-do items regarding my role as a father?"

"No," Sherrie said in a quiet voice. "I want you to just be yourself, take more time to enjoy your family, not be so uptight about doing everything for your clients or DOING things for our family. I'm suggesting you lead a simpler, more relaxed life that has fewer to-do items." Our discussion continued as we clarified issues and told each other how much we loved one another. That afternoon we tore down a few of the walls restricting the communication of our own insecurities, and were glad to have had the help of our counselor to initiate that process.

To break out of your box demands great effort and innovative thinking. Sometimes, in the midst of chronic illness or some other adversity, we just don't have the perseverance or creativity needed to bust through the walls. The wise person or couple seeks other resources to give them a helping hand or wise counsel.

My buddy John now lives in Oregon and we exchange e-mail letters at least every other day. After reading about some problem that ambushed me in 1997 he wrote a non-preachy message that included the following words. John, by the way, is the most gifted writer I know.

"Imagine being a bird, and how joyous it must be to be surprised that you can fly every time you flap your wings. If the bird doesn't suppose it should fly, then how grand whenever it does. But if you expect to fly every time you flap your wings, and do, then it becomes mundane, and small, and forgotten, even thought it's quite important. I guess this is why success gets boring (as failure must do, as well). But there is no success or failure when there's no expectation of an outcome."

Battling chronic illness sometimes seems an epic struggle against mundane failure. It takes personal effort combined with help from anywhere you can get it, be it a counselor or a friend with whom you communicate in cyberspace. It also takes a truckload of perseverance. "The foolish bird flaps his wings, nothing happens, and then never flaps them again," John wrote at the end of his letter.

One cloudy autumn day in 1997 while driving toward a consulting engagement in Fort Collins, I experienced a revelation that put John's words into perspective. On my left, a mile to the west, stood the front range of the Colorado Rocky Mountains. To the right stretched the great American desert. I've spent most of my life at the intersection of these two gargantuan geographic formations. Generally, I find them both appealing. But on this overcast day, the eastern view seemed drab and uninviting. Yet, I felt my life symbolically drifting to just such a state of cold drabness.

The pressures of coping with Sherrie's illness and many other difficulties had hurt my ability to operate my consulting business. I felt my career and family dreams were about to be dashed. For a minute I started to consider the option of closing my business and seeking gainful employment. I also thought about how Sherrie would never have any mountaintop experiences in her future. Life had me in a bear hug and it was squeezing any hope of excitement out of my days as I drove toward another boring assignment.

Then I saw a hawk floating beneath the clouds a half-mile in front of me. It rode the air with lazy, outstretched wings; a stiff wind shooting down from the peaks to the west directed its path. To me, it seemed as if life was pushing the hawk, my family and me to the flatlands of existence to the east. As the hawk crossed over the road in front of me, I whispered, "See you in the prairie, big guy." Twenty yards east of the highway, the hawk pulled a 180-degree turn, its wings flapping strongly against the wind. I pulled to the side of the road and watched the hawk going head-to-head with the gust, struggling to climb toward the mountains a mile away. It veered neither to the left nor right, it never looked back at the prairie, it climbed and soared until I lost sight of this mysterious messenger as it slipped over the top of a ridge.

It might be a minister or a counselor, a book or a sunset, that helps you break out of your box. On that day, a hawk helped me flap my wings again.

"Dig Down Deep"

— *or* —

"Unravel the Mystery"

I f you had the skills and expertise to be anything you wanted to be, what would you choose? I have a great career that wonderfully matches my skills and passion, so I cannot complain. But in my heart of hearts, I'd like to be a musician, a modern-day minstrel, singing the soft rock music of a Bruce Hornsby, David Wilcox, "Sweet Baby" James Taylor or Marc Cohn.

Music lures and inspires me because it powerfully combines words with melody and mind with heart. One of my favorite songs is a composition by Marc Cohn, the fourth selection on his 1991 album titled "Marc Cohn." To many people, the song got lost on an album that included the popular hits "Walking In Memphis" and "Silver Thunderbird." While I enjoy those two numbers, my personal "above-the-barbed-wire" theme song has become "Dig Down Deep." I have written the lyrics below, with a few thoughts from myself and others in between the verses. The lyrics sparkle with life, as Cohn, back-up vocalists and instrumentalists all "dig down deep" to bring listeners a song from the depths of the human soul.

"Dig Down Deep" by Marc Cohn

Baby let's go below the surface
See what we can find
There's no reason to be nervous
'Cause it happens all the time

In the villainous phase one of pseudo-community, relationships depend mostly on external, superficial factors. There's not much to find in our human interactions when we stay on the surface of things. From above, the ocean just looks wet and wavy. Hidden beneath that exterior is a dynamic and colorful civilization of underwater plants and animals. Likewise, when people get beyond talking about the weather and the local sports team, they often discover amazing things about each other. However, there is "reason to be nervous" because it takes courage to choose the discomfort of sharing intimate thoughts and feelings. Unfortunately, it doesn't "happen all the time" because most individuals and couples choose to stay below "the barbed wire" or (to mix metaphors) above the ocean surface.

I don't want to go up to the mountain
I don't need to go down to the sea
Gonna sit right here 'til we unravel
The mystery

We often use mindless activity as a diversion from coming face-to-face, mind-to-mind, heart-to-heart with a loved one.

To put people off we'll say things like: "We'll get together after I complete this major project." "Let's go for a walk another day. Our favorite TV shows are on tonight." "I would love to talk about how things are going with you, Junior, but I have to leave now for my parenting class." Going "up to the mountain" or "down to the sea" sounds wonderful, but it can't truly compare to the journey of going into the heart, soul and mind of a loved one, which is where you will unravel "the mystery."

> *While the lights of the city*
> *Are shining below*
> *Gonna hold onto you girl*
> *And never let go*
> *While everyone else is just walking around*
> *In their sleep*
> *Baby let's dig down*
> *Dig down deep*
> *I wanna dig down deep*

Many people not only stay above the ocean surface of relationships, they even keep their shoes and socks on when they tiptoe onto a glorious beach. They refuse to get wet, and would never consider taking a peek underwater. They are spectators at best. Those who reside in the pseudo-community phase are "just walking around" through life, destined for an emotionless mediocrity. "Baby . . . let's dig . . . down . . . deep." Let's live rather than exist, "just walking around in their [our] sleep." In his book titled *You Gotta Keep Dancin*, author and motivational speaker Tim Hansel wrote, "How can we, knowing that life is so incredibly delicious and short lived, still continue to live bland, insipid lives?" Hansel lives in ongoing pain caused by a mountain-climbing accident.

And I don't wanna wait until tomorrow
'Cause the fortune said that "The time is now"
It's time to find out what we're doing
What we're doing anyhow

Remember that we have thousands of instances when we can choose comfort or discomfort. Do I ask my loved one how he or she is doing or do I turn on some fatuous TV game show? We can "wait until tomorrow" to talk. Of course you will also face the same comfort-discomfort choice tomorrow. And what if "Sister Death" chooses to deny you tomorrow? Author Richard L. Evans wrote: "When in the world are we going to begin to live as if we understood that this is life? This is our time, our day . . . and it is passing. What are we waiting for?"

Let's go out in the moonlight
And walk for a while
Maybe stay up all night and we could
Talk for awhile
Kick off your shoes
'Cause you've got nothing to lose
But your sleep
Baby let's dig down
Dig down deep
I wanna dig down deep

While writing this essay on April 21, 1998, I asked Sherrie to have lunch with me at our kitchen table. When I sat down, she already had started eating and reading the morning's newspaper at the same time. I sat down and started to reach for another section of the paper, but stopped myself in mid-air. All of a sudden, I had made the choice to sneak through the barbed wire. "How are you doing?" I asked. For 25 minutes she explained to me that she was not doing well. "I still get so angry and depressed, never knowing from day to day whether I will be able to do much. I feel guilty having people come clean my house. I would love to take Alyse and her friends shopping in Denver tomorrow, but I know it would set me back the rest of the week," she said. I mainly listened, but found an opportunity to tell her how frustrated I felt, too. "I feel as if 'The Intruder' robs a huge portion of your freedom nearly every day. It also limits what our family can do."

A few minutes later, Sherrie shrugged and smiled, saying, "I don't hurt quite as much now just because I had a chance to gripe a little bit. Thanks for asking and listening." The conversation ended on a gentle, somewhat uplifting note but could have just as easily ended with sobs of despair. That's part of the risk – and the excitement – of "the strange and lovely ride" of discussions that "dig down deep."

It's an open invitation
So baby don't you cry
It's a life long celebration
And I think we're right on time
It's a feeling in your heart

And a lump in the throat
It's a strange and lovely ride
Wanna dig down deep inside

Don't we ever tire of the mindless, endless ride of pseudo-community? When we only deal with the superficial, when we delete emotions from life's script, we walk in partial darkness. Society might shine an angelic light on the silent martyr who is a "caretaker," but the person is actually walking in the dark while casting a shadow on those around him or her. The amazing paradox is that by communicating above the barbed wire, two or more people who struggle with ongoing difficulties might create a "lifelong celebration" seasoned with laughter and tears, trust and love, fear and sadness, joy and sorrow, peace and hope. Those are the seasonings that real, not plastic, people experience as a course of life. Chronic illness can confine individuals and couples to smaller physical spaces, but it also can be the springboard to opening new vistas in the relationship. Without even leaving the room you and your significant other can take "a strange and lovely ride" fueled by emotions and words. As Marc Cohn states it so powerfully, "dig down deep."

"Fear not that thy life will come to an end, but rather fear that it shall never have a beginning."
— Cardinal John Newman

Raising the Bar

— *or* —

Was Blind, Now I See

A s a workshop group facilitator for corporate employees, I often put my workshop participants through an exercise called, "The Blind Line." I assign them the simple task of getting into birth order by month and day (with no concern for year of birth). However, before the participants begin, I tell them to close their eyes and refrain from speaking for the duration of the exercise. These restrictions make their task possible, but extremely difficult. Only four of approximately 300 groups have successfully completed the task under these conditions.

After the group has groped and struggled for five minutes, I then have them open their eyes and tell me their thoughts and feelings. Their responses include comments such as:
- "I felt scared because I was literally in the dark."
- "I never had a sense we were working toward a common goal so our effort seemed wasted."
- "I was angry at you for giving us such a stupid assignment."
- "I felt hopeless because I knew nothing we tried would work."

In a corporate setting, I say that "The Blind Line" exercise is a metaphor for work environments. Everything participants say about the exercise could be (and has been) said about the workplace. Working in the dark – a metaphor for failing to communicate openly and honestly – prevents working effectively. If you and your loved one are "working in the dark" as you battle chronic illness, you likely feel more scared and alone than need be.

In the early part of 1996 our biggest foe shifted from Sherrie's chronic illness to difficulties involving our children. I had learned how to handle the dilemmas presented by chronic illness by talking openly about them, but amazingly I forgot how to keep open the lines of communication when dealing with other problems. A wise counselor told me once that I typically responded to stress in one of two ways: 1) I clam up and then plummet emotionally and mentally. This option presents an image of putting my hands up to prevent Sherrie and the kids from getting too close to me. 2) I become a lecturer, imparting "wisdom" to Sherrie and my children, which cuts off "dig down deep" communication. This option is akin to a painful bear hug that overwhelms those around me, preventing them from responding in an open and truthful way.

This counselor suggested I try to implement a third option, between the two extremes above, with regard to how I deal with stress. A gentle, loving squeeze represents this healthy option. It involves encouraging others to speak from the heart, to listen without judging, to share my own emotional responses, to guide, rather than direct.

In my workshops with corporate employees, after the first "Blind Line" discussion, I have the group again line up, shoulder to shoulder. I tell them I want them to get into birth order. "Are there any questions?"

"Um, can we talk and open our eyes?"

"You bet," I say.

"Which end is January and which is December?"

I tell them. Then I let them begin. It usually takes 20 seconds or less to complete the task "with the lights on." The group participants' IQs did not magically increase between the first and second versions of the activity. What happened is that I created an open, rather than closed environment. In other words, clarity brings power – whether in a corporate or family setting.

During a counseling session in 1996, Sherrie described how alone she felt at times. I figured she felt alone because chronic illness prevented her from working, which meant she spent many hours in an empty house each day. Unlike me, our counselor, Roy, chose to clarify, rather than assume, what she meant. "Why do you feel so alone, Sherrie?"

"Because Gregg has become so distant," she said.

I sat in shock as Sherrie talked for five minutes about the emotional barrier she felt I had erected between us. In her eyes, Sherrie believed that the barrier created by my distance prevented us from improving our relationship and helping our children work through tough times.

"What do you want from Gregg?" Roy asked, as I remained silent. She looked at me and said, "I want you to schedule me into your life." In a fraction of a second, I became "Mr. Time Manager," thinking of ways to plug her into the ol' DayTimer. Roy stepped in quickly. "I don't want to put words in your mouth, Sherrie, but I don't think that's really what you want from Gregg." That dullard part of me that longs for the comfort of pseudo-community whispered inside my head, "Uh-oh."

"You want Gregg to place you in his heart," Roy said as he shifted his gaze from Sherrie to me. My wife nodded silently while her eyes also turned to me. Roy had raised the bar significantly in that one sentence. I could put Sherrie into my DayTimer while still residing as a martyred "caretaker" dwelling in the pseudo-community phase. I could wear the label, operate in the dark, stay above the ocean surface, wear shoes and socks on the beach, be a tough John "the Duke" Wayne and schedule her into my life. But to truly place her in my heart meant to go above the barbed wire, shed the "caretaker" label, communicate in the light, go below the surface, let the sand massage my toes, and gun down the independent, stoical figure of "the Duke."

The room grew quiet and I soon sensed Roy and Sherrie would not open their mouths again until after I responded, even if it took a minute, a day or a decade. My mind raced for 30 seconds – which seemed like 30 minutes – as I sought for the right words of reply. Then my heart slipped into the control chair while my muddled brain took a break.

"I'm empty," I said in a voice that was barely audible. "I don't know how to put you into my heart, Sherrie." And in that apparently weak (but vulnerable) and confused (but honest) answer, I began the next leg of my journey with my wife toward the community of phase four.

"That's OK," Sherrie said with sincerity. "I'm not sure how to do it either, but I know we can figure it out."

Country and Western musician (and occasional philosopher) Garth Brooks sings, "Life is not about a finish line, it's about a chase." Sometimes I pull off to the side of the road on this journey toward lifelong community. I grow weary or stupid, falling back on old phase-one habits. But in the whole scheme of things, Sherrie and I continue to progress down the road of life, sometimes dragging our dusty sandals, sometimes kicking up our heels in joy, never fully surrendering, striving toward a finish line unseen and unreachable, but worthy of the chase.

chapter 11

THE "BIG 5" IN
PHASE FOUR

There are many different ways to fight back
against "The Intruder."

Support:
Adapt Your Mindset

— or —

Third-Down and Four-to-Go

A football team loses its strong-armed quarterback to injury and the coach switches his focus from a passing to a running attack. A corporation sells one of its manufacturing operations to another company, and the latter must change its focus from that of a cost center (with internal, captive customers) to that of a profit center (which must aggressively win external customers). An international conglomerate transfers an American manager and her family to England. The cultural rules that impact her family change overnight.

The examples above are different and similar at the same time. The connection between each can be summed up in one word: adaptation. The adaptations required of each of the scenarios above are as follows: On a crucial third-down and with four yards to go, the coach calls for a running play instead of a passing play. The manufacturing operation evaluates itself by a profit-and-loss sheet rather than how well it matches arbitrary goals developed by an unnamed manager at company headquarters and the American manager and her family learn to drive on the left side of the road instead of the right.

When chronic illness ambushes a family like mine, the "rules of life" change. What used to be common – Mom going for daily five-mile runs or the family taking an expensive vacation during Spring Break – becomes uncommon or impossible. The paradox of it all is that some people believe that adapting to the changing circumstances is surrendering to the enemy, chronic illness in my family's case.

Let's examine the football example again. In professional sports, team owners evaluate coaches primarily by their win/ loss record. If the coach continues to rely on the passing attack when his new quarterback is scatter-armed at best, that is surrendering to the enemy. To adapt his play selection is not a surrender, but a wise, progressive strategy for improving the odds of victory. As I was writing this essay, I saw Ann, a friend of ours who cleans houses to help supplement her family's income, scrubbing the kitchen floor. For three hours every week, Ann comes in to help Sherrie and me clean our house. When Sherrie and I were growing up, professional house cleaners never passed through our front doors. Our mothers, with the help of their families, did their own cleaning, thank you very much. And we came into our adulthood thinking the same way. However, that philosophy changed when Sherrie got sick. At first Sherrie and I both felt somewhat guilty having Ann scrub our toilets, vacuum our carpets and dust our furniture. We don't anymore, because we are merely adapting to current circumstances.

We pay Ann a few bucks for cleaning our house each week. If we decided to save those few bucks we give her, I would have to clean the house which would keep me from the many activities I do to earn a living. Instead of resting her weary body, gathering strength for when the kids arrive from school, were Ann not available, Sherrie might be irritating her already sore hips by having to clean the bathroom mirrors. Oh, Sherrie still does plenty of household chores on a weekly basis, but Ann does the heavy-duty stuff, leaving us more time and energy for activities we can do ourselves.

You might not be able to afford housecleaning services. Even if you can, it just might seem too much of a luxury to spend on yourself or a loved one. Perhaps you need to adjust your mindset if that's the case. If your loved one needs headache medicine, you find a way to pay for it. If he or she needs to go in for a medical check-up, you write out a check. Sherrie and I are looking for any and all options that will help us live successfully with chronic illness. Over the years, the frugal part of me has become more willing to invest in house-cleaning services, recliner chairs and matinee tickets, among other things, convincing myself these things fell in the same category as doctor and prescription expenses. Perhaps you still struggle with spending money on what you consider frivolous items. If you are a classic "caretaker" you will solve the problem by adding more "duties" to your already busy life. If your significant other can't clean the house then, by gum, you'll do it yourself, in between times of earning wages 60 hours a week and handling the bulk of the parenting challenges.

If you get nothing else from this book, I hope you understand you need to take care of yourself. Someone in your life has a body that is crashing and burning to some extent. The last thing your relationship or family needs is two unhealthy bodies – be they emotionally, mentally or physically impaired.

If you can afford a house cleaner or a new recliner chair or occasional matinee movie tickets (or whatever is important to your loved one and you) then pay for them. That money is an investment in your health, rather than money thrown away for luxuries. If you shift your mindset it becomes easier to funnel the money in that direction.

But what if you flat-out don't have discretionary funds for such items? If that's the case, discover more creative ways to adapt. Maybe you decide to boost your children's allowances while adding more household responsibilities to their daily chores. Maybe you'll have to agree that the family will survive just fine, even if the house is not shiny bright and germ free. Maybe you decide not to take that trip to Mexico this Spring Break, but go to a guest ranch on the outskirts of your own town instead. Adaptation is a key to maintaining some sense of control and victory over chronic illness. Adapt your mindset; convince yourself and your significant other that what used to be frivolous expenditures are now wise investments in your fight against "The Intruder." It's third-and-four in the game of life. What play are you going to call?

Medical Maze:
Nose to the Carpet

— or —

Fighter or Victim?

You walk into your house one sunny afternoon with no fear of impending disaster. This house is your safe domain. In a world gone crazy, this is your castle of tranquility, the one spot in the world where you can let down your guard and get away from it all. You set your house keys down on the counter and then a huge fist smacks the back of your neck. The next thing you know, you are face down on the ground with an intruder snarling threats in your ear.

Fortunately, burglars and thugs have never entered my home. People who have been burglarized feel as if the thieves physically violated them even if the robbery occurred in their absence. These homeowners never regain their previous sense of security, even in their houses. In a sense, chronic illness does the same thing. In the light of day – when life seems as safe and serene as a fortified, beloved abode – sickness strikes unsuspecting individuals and those who love them. One day you walk boldly down the hallway of life, and the next second you're face down, with your nose scrunched against the carpet.

The illness itself is the thug who pins you against the floor. However, unseen accomplices may be part of this conniving team as well. Maybe it's a doctor with the bedside manner of an IRS auditor, or insurance company officials with the generosity of – well – insurance company officials. You can be the meekest person on the block and still want to fight back against the thug pressing his foul body against a loved one or yourself. If chronic illness magically became a person for the day, Sherrie and I would both attack the culprit, aiming for the vulnerable spots on the thug's body. Alas, the core of Sherrie's chronic illness is as invisible and elusive as the deadly fumes of carbon monoxide.

But the accomplices are another matter. Most of the "accomplices" to chronic illness (that Sherrie and I have known) have been human beings – although their actions sometimes make you wonder about their humanity. I'm not suggesting you corner a doctor while brandishing a scalpel from his drawer or proposing you hire a hit man to bonk the kneecaps of your friendly insurance rep. I am stating, however, that there can be emotional benefit in standing up to the "accomplices."

In early 1998, Corlet and Alyse participated in a one-day "Model Mugging" workshop. This program teaches verbal and physical methods for warding off would-be assailants. During the closing ceremony, the 14 participants showed off their newfound skills to the amazement of their parents, grandparents and friends. You could see the emotional release each of the participants experienced by pounding on well-padded male "assailants." The girls talked of feeling empowered and fearless from attending the workshop as they walked out of the building. Unfortunately, "patients" and "caretakers" rarely get a chance to savor the feelings of release and empowerment, especially if they behave according to their labels. Somewhere along the line, however, Sherrie and I started changing our approach to how we dealt with chronic illness, becoming less nice and polite and more assertive and empowered.

During a hospital stay in 1992, our insurance company sought to have Sherrie discharged before we felt she was ready. Maybe you can't fight city hall, but you can fight insurance companies. While still in the hospital she contacted medical professionals willing to speak on her behalf. She insisted an insurance rep drive 90 minutes from Denver to the hospital to meet with her and the medical team. She looked the representative in the eyes and told him she planned to stay in the hospital for another few days and expected him to support that decision. Her conviction, along with the advice and support of her team of doctors, persuaded the representative to approve her request. And for a few days, Sherrie felt as if she had loosened the grip of "The Intruder's" choke hold.

In late 1996, a semi-truck hit our van after Sherrie stopped at a stop sign. The truck driver's insurance company refused to assume any responsibility for the accident. Well, there's nothing to do about that, right? If you are a wimpy, stoical "victim," then that statement is true. Since Sherrie would never consider herself to be a victim, she chose a different course of action. Although it took time, energy and money, Sherrie chose to file a lawsuit against the trucking company. She had to testify in a pre-trial deposition, withstanding tough questions from lawyers. But the expertise of our attorney, combined with Sherrie's decision to stand firm, earned her an out-of-court settlement. It was not a six-figure-we-are-now-filthy-rich settlement, but it definitely covered medical expenses and boosted our children's college fund. More importantly, it again gave Sherrie a chance to fight back, regaining some control and self-respect.

Remember, my goal in life used to be to have everyone like me. I felt comfortable in the pseudo-community phase where people are nice and polite and sweep conflict under the rug. Thanks to my long acquaintance with chronic illness, I have been able to burst out of the box created by phase one. I have been willing to tell a doctor over the phone what I really think of his worthless diagnosis, and I have supported Sherrie when she takes unpopular and uncomfortable stands in her fight against accomplices. I do not suggest you fight your "Intruder" and its accomplices in the same manner Sherrie and I fought ours. But I strongly recommend you fight back by trashing the labels, communicating openly and seeking personal and relational growth. Will you be a victim or a fighter?

Parenting:
Unpopular but Right

— *or* —

The Good Side of Being Selfish

I opened up the local newspaper and saw the headline about a rare murder in Loveland. Then I noticed the photograph of a man and woman being led in shackles through a court-house hallway. They were the parents of one of Bret's best friends. The headline and photograph started a new chapter of my family's life during 1996. My 7-year-old son knew the victim and the murderers who had confessed. The man who was killed had been a roommate of his slayers. Bret never spent the night at his friend's house, but had spent several hours in the home in the 18 months leading up to the crime. Obviously, explaining the murder to my young son proved challenging.

Sherrie and I wondered if anything bad had ever happened to Bret on his visits. His friend, I'll call him Jim, spent days and days playing at our house. We wondered if Jim had known about the murder committed in his house, and whether he had told his little buddy Bret about his "secret." Later, after the parents were convicted and sent to prison, we found out Jim had come upon the scene of the crime shortly after the killing. We also found out later that Bret had seen red splotches on the dining room wall, carpets and stairs and had been told they were stains from spilt Hawaiian Punch. It was no wonder that Bret had been sullen and explosive in recent weeks, Sherrie and I thought.

One day, shortly after Jim and his sister (I'll call her Brenda) started living in a local foster home, Sherrie, Bret and I took a walk through the neighborhood. Midway through the autumn excursion, Bret said, "Mom and I want to talk to you and the girls about adopting Jim and Brenda." I nodded but said: "Let's not talk to the girls about that yet. We're not even sure that will be an option and I need to think a long time about the situation." Two days later Sherrie and I sat in our counselor's office. I told Sherrie and Roy that I had had many thoughts as we walked home two nights earlier.

"I felt as if I had to be a martyr working long hours to pay for college for five kids," I said. "I imagined trying to find time to be the perfect, supportive father of a huge clan. I also felt great rage against Jim's so-called parents who shattered many lives through their murderous act." Roy and Sherrie listened.

"By the time we got home that night," I continued, "I felt as if I wore a hundred-pound cloak of responsibility."

My words proved to be a springboard to more open and honest discussion between Sherrie and me. Roy summarized our conversation by saying that Sherrie felt great compassion for the kids and I felt overwhelming responsibility when I thought of adoption. We agreed to keep talking about the issue in the weeks ahead. In reality, though, we let the topic stew on the back burner for a while. Six weeks later, on Nov. 5, 1996, the foster mother called Sherrie to ask if we would be willing to adopt Jim and Brenda. She said the brother and sister hoped to become part of our family. When Sherrie told me about the call, she made the possibility sound glorious. I, on the other hand, felt as if Evander Holyfield had given me an uppercut to the gut. I felt scared and told her so.

"I appreciate your honesty," Sherrie replied. Even as she spoke those words I sensed she despised my outlook. I felt backed into a corner: damned if I adopt and damned if I don't. Six days later, Jim and Brenda accompanied us to church, after which we all went out to eat lunch. Jim and Brenda were bright kids who had lived in a bleak environment. My heart softened toward them and I came close to saying aloud that we should adopt them. Sherrie was poised for me to say it and ready to leap into action when I did. But I remembered the puppy incident of four years before. You can take an unwanted puppy back to the pound, but you can't do the same with kids. I feared I would do all the fatherly duties, but would quietly bitch and moan about my stressful life for decades to come, making everyone as miserable as myself.

A few more days passed and Sherrie continued to play it cool. I constantly thought about the topic. I wrote about the pros and cons of the adoption in my journal and I also sought advice from people I trusted, who fell into either the "You guys are angelic" or "You guys are crazy" camps. The old Gregg Piburn classified Sherrie as compassionate and myself as selfish. Many times I came close to making the "unselfish" and "popular" decision to adopt. But like a young soldier afraid to fire the first shot in battle, I kept my trigger finger ready, but still. I considered the impact of adding another pair of kids to the three children we already have. My mind thought of advantages and disadvantages. Bret was gung-ho on the idea, while the girls – 14 and 15 at the time – had far more important middle-school matters on their mind.

I kept hoping an answer from above would come to me like a flash of lightning, but it didn't. I tried to remember my night-time dreams for a clue about what do to. The more I thought about it, the heavier the cloak of responsibility felt. The more I sought the answer, the more muddled my thinking became. Then one day, while walking alone in the neighborhood, the answer came in a simple phrase that stuck in my brain.

"I don't want to do it."
The musty cloak slipped from my back
"I ... don't ... want ... to ... do ... it."

That night, after the kids were in bed, I sat in the family room with Sherrie. "I've come to a decision about whether to adopt Jim and Brenda," I told Sherrie. She listened quietly as I said, "I don't want to do it." Perhaps that is all I would have needed to say in a perfect world, but I explained some of my reasons. "We have plenty of stress in this family without adding more. It is not our job to save every person in the world who has a problem. I worry about the financial burden it will put on us. I think adopting two kids would prevent us from giving Corlet, Alyse and Bret the attention they need and deserve. But mainly, Sherrie, I just don't want to do it."

She thanked me for being honest and confessed she had started having doubts about the wisdom of adding two more children to the family. However, two or three more times over the next week Sherrie slipped the thought of adoption into the conversation. The third time I said quietly, but firmly,

"How many times, in how many ways do I have to tell you, I don't want to do it?"

Sherrie finally read the message loud and clear. Later on she told me she felt good about my decision, our decision. Then she called the foster mother to say we could not adopt Jim and Brenda. A few times in the past two years Sherrie has told me: "I am so thankful we didn't bring two more kids into our family. I don't think we could have handled it."

Today, Jim and Brenda live in another state with new parents. I trust they are fine and better off not having a miserable, stressed-out father like me in their lives. One night, not long after we decided not to add to our family through adoption, I watched a TV commercial for the YMCA that showed a 77-year-old volunteer who plays basketball with and mentors troubled young men. "If you have a positive impact on two or three people in your life, you have done a good job," the man said at the end of the ad.

We did not adopt Jim and Brenda but, based on the wise volunteer's math, I have done a good job with my life. The keys to my success are many, but the ones that stand out the most have been my willingness to strip the confining label of "caretaker" off my back, to have the courage to stand up and say what I want and what I don't want, and to have the wisdom to understand that doing both things does not necessarily mean I am selfish or evil.

Intimacy:
Walking a Tightrope

— *or* —

Commitment Is Freedom

About three years into Sherrie's illness, Vance, a co-worker of mine, told me of his marital problems. I mainly listened to him, but since I had 15 years of marital experience under my belt, Vance asked my advice about how he could save his marriage. To help Vance out, I suggested that he and his wife, Sue, first make a commitment to stay married. If they did that, I said, they would have the foundation upon which to build a firm relationship. Unfortunately, commitment does not guarantee a lasting marriage, but I strongly believe it increases a couples' odds of staying together. Every time I mentioned this tack, Vance looked dumbfounded for a few seconds. Then he would say something such as, "Sue and I love our personal freedom too much to tie ourselves down to such a long-term arrangement." To Vance commitment meant confinement, a loss of freedom.

One night Vance and Sue came over to have dinner with Sherrie and me and we talked about how to save their marriage. In the living room after the kids had gone to bed, Sue asked Sherrie what she needed to do to strengthen her relationship with Vance.

"First you must be committed to each other and the marriage," Sherrie said. "Without that commitment, I'm not sure there's much else to do to save the relationship." Like her short-sighted husband, Sue balked at the idea of a heartfelt commitment.

"To me," said Sue, who had been married three or four times, "commitment ties me down too much. I love Vance, but I don't want us to have to make such a scary commitment to each other." In other words, for Sue also, commitment meant confinement. A few days later Vance caught me at work and told me he had argued with Sue the previous night. "I don't even know if she will be home when I get to my house tonight," he said with panic in his voice. "If she is there, I know I'll have to watch every word I say. We have gone through this before and if I say the wrong thing she will split – for a day, for a week, forever."

I listened intently to his words and replied nonjudgmentally. But I wondered how his "non-commitment" marriage equated to freedom. Vance sounded as if he dwelled on a verbal tightrope, afraid to say the wrong words for fear of causing the final break-up. To Vance, mere arguments took on a whole new dimension because a few mispoken words could be the fatal slip that sent the couple plunging to marital death.

Vance and Sue believed commitment meant loss of freedom. Society effectively peddles that message for this and many other couples. In an ironic twist on society's message, I believe commitment brings freedom. Obviously, I advocate open and honest communication in a marriage. But if I had been in Vance's shoes, afraid that one verbal misstep could lead to long-term break-up, I would also have chosen my words carefully, most likely keeping some of the "lights off" in my discussions with an on-edge spouse.

Sherrie and I, however, have committed to a lifetime together, which means that words, even when spoken in anger, do not represent threats to the relationship. We can say and do many things openly without fear of it leading to divorce. This, by the way, does not mean we can say or do anything. If I'm unfaithful to Sherrie or start punching her out, I believe she has reason to consider a divorce. However, short of those huge errors in judgment, we have the freedom to share our feelings, offer our suggestions and spill our guts. Since we have signed up for the long haul, we might as well use all our resources to work things out for the best. In the midst of a complex society, a complex relationship (which all marriages are) deserves open and honest discussion.

This issue of maintaining a lifelong relationship is especially relevant in marriages affected by chronic illness. The American divorce rate hovers around 50 percent. However, in marriages where one of the partners is chronically ill, the divorce rate zooms to 75 percent, according to Sefra Kobrin Pitzele in her book titled *We Are Not Alone: Learning to Live with Chronic Illness.*

Chronic illness obviously puts a strain on a relationship. It forces couples to adapt (not an easy chore for most) or it brings them crashing down if they try to maintain the lifestyle they had before a partner became ill. The strain is especially onerous if "caretakers" play by the rules of their label. One key to keeping a marriage or relationship alive is for the "caretaker" to trash the label and associated duties ascribed to the term. Another key is to make a commitment to the relationship. Both keys open up the lines of communication, a critical element in any relationship, especially one coming face-to-face with a formidable foe such as chronic illness.

Most couples who have gone through a wedding ceremony have made a public commitment to their relationship. Unfortunately, that commitment (contained within the vows) seemingly means little to many people who fail to live up to them. Cartoonist Wiley Miller hit it on the head when he drew a wedding scene for his one-panel comic strip titled, "Non Sequitur." Under the heading "Modern Commitment," the caption read: ". . . And with this ring, I vow to give it a shot. But I'm not promising anything."

On Aug. 19, 1973, Sherrie and I received a special gift from Rev. Eugene Allen, who had performed our wedding ceremony minutes before. He gave us a script of our entire wedding, written in his beautiful penmanship. Here are the words of our vows.

"I, Gregg, take you, Sherrie, to be my wedded wife; and I do promise and covenant, before God and these witnesses, to be your loving and faithful husband, in plenty and in want, in joy and in sorrow, in health and in sickness, as long as we both shall live." Sherrie made the same declaration and we have lived up to that promise. But don't get the idea we've stayed together simply out of obligation to some spoken words.

A friend named Andy pruned one of our trees in the mid-'90s. The fallen branches from the trees reminded me of broken marriages, heaped high in the post-sexual revolution of the 1960s. On the way home, Andy, who is a college professor, said: "I know several couples who have struggled with chronic illness. You and Sherrie are the only two who have stuck together. For some reason, I would not have picked the two of you as the ones who would have remained married. Why do you think you are still together?"

When Andy asks a question, it usually demands several seconds of thought and then a lengthy reply. This time, however, I answered quickly and succinctly. "That's easy. I have always loved Sherrie and know I always will." That was not a politically correct answer. It was as true as I could be. I loved Sherrie when she was a young, vivacious woman who had picked the same sort of lifestyle I chose and I love her even more since seeing her respond to a life with fewer options.

In his book *Mystery of Marriage*, Mike Mason wrote: "For marriage involves nothing more than a lifelong commitment to love just one person – to do, whatever else one does, a good, thorough job of loving one person. What could be simpler than that? There is nothing simpler than love." Two things "The Intruder" cannot rob from us is our love for and commitment to each other. In those things, we maintain freedom, blessed freedom.

Spiritual:
Down from the Pedestal

— *or* —

The Dream Message

In the summer of 1965, at the age of 14, I decided I didn't ever have to die. Despite having many friends, mainly teammates on various sports teams, I was a loner who spent many hours pondering weighty issues. That particular summer, I determined I had the mind and body to overcome death. One evening my parents sat in the front seat and I in the back as we drove 20 miles to my aunt and uncle's house. The Colorado Rocky Mountains loomed over us less than a mile from the car window.

What if, I thought, this car drove off a winding mountain road and plunged into a canyon hundreds of feet below? I figured that my well-trained mind would determine the exact moment, just before impact, when my well-trained body should jump up and out of the car. The car would crash into smithereens, but I would hit the ground as if stepping off the bottom rung of a step ladder. Such was the heady thinking of a young teenager growing up in Boulder, Colo., in the 1960s with a Pony League baseball championship under his belt. If I could be the winning pitcher over mighty Twinburger in the title game, then I could surely defeat The Grim Reaper.

Obviously, my 14-year-old philosophy on life and death needed major reconstruction. More than three decades later, I'm positive The Grim Reaper (or, more to my liking, "Sister Death") will end my mortal, earthly life. Even though my philosophy had many holes, it represented the spiritual part of my life to some extent. If asked, most people would say they are physical beings who happen to have a spiritual component. However, there is a small percentage who would be prone to admit that they are spiritual beings who happen to have a physical component.

If we asked 100 people to describe the spiritual element of life, we would probably get 100 different answers. When I try to describe it, words such as intangible, limitless, critically important and eternal in nature come to mind. To me, spirituality deals with an individual's perspective on, among other things, creation, God and eternity – important issues that lack black-and-white answers. These issues encompass time, space and mental capacities we can't fathom.

Part of the spiritual equation, however, has less to do with light years and Supreme Beings than it does with the here and now . . . and you. Who are you and why are you here? Most of us rarely, if ever, ponder that question. It is much easier to get caught up in a championship season or the latest career opportunity than in such a thought-provoking question. Yet, in our unknown and unseeing way, we try to answer that question. In 1965, I knew I was at my best on the baseball field and could live through a death-defying crash in the mountains. That "knowledge" was part of my spiritual component.

However, our view of ourselves changes dramatically as our lives change. At times I've traded in my never-say-die attitude of 1965 to a get-me-out-of-here defensive posture. After giving a presentation, I might receive 10 compliments and one mild criticism. My brain latches onto the critical comment, forgetting the compliments. These viewpoints help determine – at any moment – who I am and why I'm here. At times, I have beat myself up for being the physically healthy person in my marriage. At times, I have felt guilty for being angry at Sherrie or the illness. My self-esteem often plummets if I fail to live up to my unrealistic standards as a husband, father, consultant and friend. At times, I have believed I deserved a quick death and gloomy eternity.

The montage of events, interactions and learnings from your days creates the self-image that helps define your spiritual life. It comes from a combination of living through a crisis, or hearing what others think about you, or reading a powerful book. In 1997 a clue to who I am and why I'm here came to me in a different way – a dream. I don't usually remember dreams. Occasionally I will recall snippets of distorted images that have murky, if any, meaning. However, one night, while in the midst of another difficult period of my life, I got a new glimpse of myself through a dream.

I have one brother and no sisters. Mike is nearly eight years older than I am. I have always been the type of kid brother who looks at his sibling in awe, even now when we are both middle-aged. My vision of him as a big brother creates unrealistic expectations of him as a person. Nobody could live up to the picture I have of my brother. In remembrances of the dreams I have had, Mike often makes cameo appearances, even though in reality, I only see him for about four days each year. In this particular dream I am standing in a stark, white-walled room. I look to my left and see a figure standing alone, looking away from me at the wall. I peer long and hard at the figure, who is wearing khaki pants and a denim shirt, as I try to determine who he is. Eventually, the distant figure looks quickly my way and then back at the wall. Well, what do you know, I thought, it's Mike.

In my dream, I take a few hesitant steps toward my brother. I have the sense I can speak to him if I want to, but I choose to remain quiet, like a mountain lion stalking a deer. Every few seconds I take another step or two toward the figure. My unrealistic expectations of Mike peel away with each step I take. As I draw nearer, I start to see the figure in a different light. He is no longer my "big brother," standing like a giant in my little-kid eyes. He is just a man, my height, middle-aged, who as a longtime husband, father, breadwinner and friend, has battled his share of crises – some big, some small. I see the image in my dream as a man who has a wonderful relationship with a great wife. Yet, his shoulders droop a little, hardly the posture of a kingly brother. I see the image in my dream as a man who has helped raise two sons into semi-crazy, but glorious manhood. But despite that victory, he has streaks of gray in his hair.

Then I realize that I love Mike even more when I view him as a real man, stepped down from the pedestal I put him on decades before. He didn't have to live up to my impossible standards and he didn't seem a failure if he didn't. Now, I stand within an arm's reach of my brother. More than anything, I want to give him a strong hug that expresses my great love and admiration for this man who has lived a good, difficult and normal life. It was not to be a quick parting hug with the obligatory three pats on the back that we give each other on holidays. This was to be a hug that spoke of love and respect.

In my dream I pull my brother into my arms, his head going between my head and shoulder. We hug long and hard in true brotherly fashion, devoid of any dreamy, sexual connotations. My hug is a tribute to a mere man who has fought the good fight. After a few seconds, we slowly pull away from each other. Then I see the face. It's similar to my brother's, but it doesn't carry his countenance. The face I look into is mine.

chapter 12

FINDING
YOUR VOICE

Fighting a mysterious and insidious illness
is difficult. It is nearly impossible if you are
mysterious and insidious yourself. See how
important it is to get a handle on who you are.

Quiet Desperation

— *or* —

Voices Set Free

R obin Williams portrayed prep-school English teacher John Keating in the movie "Dead Poets Society." In a classic scene, Keating stands on his desk to help students understand the importance of seeing things from different perspectives. Then he has each boy spend a few seconds atop his desk. Looking up at the students on their desks, Keating tells the group, "Boys, you must strive to find your own voice." Moments later he adds, "Thoreau said, 'Most men lead lives of quiet desperation.'" I believe people impacted by chronic illness might learn something from those two statements.

First, what does Keating mean by voice? It's a writer's term. For example, if contemporary author John Grisham wrote his version of Hemingway's *The Old Man and the Sea*, most readers would clearly be able to tell the difference between the two books. Grisham and Hemingway's distinctive voices would be evident through the choice of words written on each page, even if the plots were identical. A great writer emits the essence of who he or she is through their words written on paper.

But what about the voices of non-writers? I believe the elements of a person's voice include personal philosophies, skills and interests. It is expressing the real you in real life. If you can't express those elements, your voice is muffled. And if you go through life with a muffled voice, it's easy to see why you might lead a "life of quiet desperation." It is the quiet desperation of a bird caged in a pet store. It is the quiet desperation of an athlete on crutches watching from the sidelines. It is the quiet desperation of a brilliant artist in a corporate cubicle producing business graphs for overhead slides.

Anyone who has dealt with chronic illness directly or indirectly knows it creates a major detour in the lives of those affected. Going from a smooth four-lane highway to a bumpy two-lane country road forces you to drive differently. Similarly, chronic illness forces you to live differently. The challenge of dealing with chronic illness involves adapting your life without risking the loss of your voice. To help clarify what I mean, here are some of the elements of my voice and how I sought to express them in the midst of Sherrie's conditions.

1. Risk taker. I chose to take a career risk despite Sherrie's illness, which made us a one-income family. Becoming my own boss in a one-person business was the best career decision of my life. It set me free and let my voice sing. This risk paid off for me in greater self-esteem and more energy to battle "The Intruder."

2. Real. I finally realized that to be a "caretaker" in the pseudo-community phase was counter-productive. More than ever, Sherrie needed to know that the real me was truly by her side. We opened up our relationship as we opened up our lines of communication.

3. Learning and teaching philosophy. In Chapter 9, I wrote about a career philosophy: "Whatever happens, use it as a learning and teaching opportunity." In my personal life, I finally learned the truth that real growth comes in times of trial. The issues surrounding chronic illness have been tough but wise instructors. By taking this philosophy out of moth balls, it brought many new lessons for my family and me.

4. OK to be disliked. I discovered it was permissible to be assertive and, at times acerbic, with medical and insurance professionals. I also found it relieved some of the stress created by chronic illness when I allowed myself to torque off other people in my life. To me, being the polite and stoical "caretaker" plays right into the hands of chronic illness. Letting my voice of being disliked express itself is one way to fight back against "The Intruder."

Chronic illness forces many people to give up many things. One thing you must strive to maintain, however, is your voice – it is one of your best weapons against "The Intruder."

The Productivity Patrol

— or —

The Unplanned Meeting

Zooming south from Fort Collins to Loveland at slightly above the speed limit, I glanced down at my daily calendar like a pirate scanning a treasure map. Whoa, I thought to myself, I have 90 minutes before my next meeting at 4 p.m. The year was 1987, two years into Sherrie's illness. At that time of my life I felt that the daily calendar was my personal owner's manual. It told me how to assemble each day, what to do and when to do it. It served as the anchor and compass of my being, even as I struggled to keep my career and family afloat.

As I eased up on the accelerator, my jammed briefcase – propped open in the back seat – caught my attention. It was a visual reminder of several impending deadlines I had to meet. At that second, I would have traded all of those responsibilities, along with my salary and benefits, for a month of peaceful existence devoid of chronic illness and daily calendars.

Enough of that foolishness! Like a cursor scanning a disk directory, my brain considered several options for how to spend the next 90 minutes. One compartment of the briefcase contained materials for a partnership project, while another section held notes for a press release. A book on writing peeked out from the back compartment, in case I ever found a few minutes for light reading. As I traveled toward

Loveland on that sunny afternoon, another option popped into my head. Why not buzz home for 30 minutes to surprise my wife and daughter? "But wait," I told myself, "if I spend 30 minutes on project planning today, it will free up a half-hour for productive work tomorrow." Such thinking is widespread in the corporate world and it obviously had affected me, judging by the way I was thinking. Earlier that year, I saw a sign above a co-worker's desk that read: "My goal is to be productive every second of the day." My mind rebelled at that philosophy, but my behavior hinted I was a potential recruit to the productivity patrol.

My foot instinctively pressed down on the accelerator as my brain mapped out directions to the public library where I could set up shop before the 4 p.m. meeting. Just as I prepared to pass a motorist with the gall to travel at the speed limit, I envisioned an Ashleigh Brilliant quote that hangs on my office wall: "If nothing's pursuing me, and nothing's waiting for me, why am I in such a hurry?" Again, I eased up on the pedal. Even my pulse seemed to downshift as I finally determined my destination – home. I hoped to see Sherrie's face light up with joy at my surprise visit, but felt disappointed when the first thing she said was: "Glad you're home. I have to pick up Corlet from school and run an errand. Alyse is napping and I'll be back in 30 minutes." The door closed and I stood in the middle of the living room on a Monday afternoon with nothing to do until my next meeting. I felt as if every time-management guru who ever lived looked at me with ghastly disdain for the poor choice I had made.

The challenges and responsibilities of coping with chronic illness could easily fill up a briefcase or two. Some weeks it seemed that dealing with Sherrie's illness sapped all of our thoughts and energy. We fed, clothed and sheltered our two daughters, but probably failed to give them the focused attention they wanted and needed. I drifted to my desk, again grasping for something useful to do for a few precious moments. If nothing else, I thought, I could tap out my daily journal entry. As I sat down at my desk, I saw movement out of the corner of my eye. My reed-thin, 5-year-old daughter, Alyse, stood in the adjacent room, blanket in hand and thumb firmly inserted in her mouth. She wore the look of a zombie – the same expression I wear when I awaken. Through the years I have learned it's useless to talk to Alyse when she's so recently been in dreamland. After a 10-second stare-down, she quietly curled up on a nearby couch, her round eyes open wide and her mouth still clamped around her thumb.

Then, despite the fact it was not on my to-do list, I made the wisest time-management decision of the day. I walked into the room, gently squeezed in beside Alyse on the couch, and cradled her in my arms without saying a word. Our slow, synchronized breathing mingled with the soft sounds of leaves shuffling in the breeze outside. I closed my eyes and hoped time would stop. I blotted from my mind the helter-skelter activity of the day and the hieroglyphics of my tattered daily calendar. In place of these visions, I painted a picture in my mind of a sometimes-too-busy father engulfing his daughter with love. I imprinted on my mind the way it felt to hold a beloved little daughter next to my body on a workday afternoon. I knew Alyse would forget the specifics of this day, but hoped she would magically carry for a lifetime the sense of love and security she must have felt at that moment.

After 10 minutes, the sound of the garage door opening interrupted our silent, unplanned meeting. Corlet burst into the room, first-grade papers spilling out of her backpack. Alyse bolted from my arms. The two little sisters dashed down the hallway to be productive at play (the one thing that would be on their to-do list if they had one). Sherrie went to the kitchen to plan the night's menu, and I slowly walked to the car where my lonely briefcase stood. I hated leaving home for a boring meeting, but I felt rejuvenated, as if Alyse had filled my tank with her innocence and potential.

"Our life is frittered away by detail . . . simplify, simplify!" wrote Henry David Thoreau. Nowadays, I write with pencil rather than pen in my daily calendar and (dare I say?) some days I fail to open it up at all. Those are the moments when I feel like simply riding the waves of the day, free from the constraints of schedules, destinations, to-do lists and labels.

One Label that Works

— *or* —

Imperfections & Journeys

O ur adopted son, Bret, classifies his ethnicity as African-American-Swedish, a lengthy and accurate statement. Blatant bigotry has bypassed Bret so far in his short life. One day at the park, however, an older schoolboy called him "the black kid." It seemingly did not bother Bret significantly, but it reminded me of how labels put a box around us.

Much of this book is about how living up to the nefarious labels of "caretaker" and "patient" harm individuals and relationships. In Chapter 2, I wrote an essay titled "Sticky Labels, Mental Chains *or* Be Set Free." If you recall, I had attendees at my presentation brainstorm roles and personalities for jobs labeled "caretaker" and "patient." They came up with the following lists.

PATIENT	CARETAKER
Depressed	Burdened
Restricted	A saint
Whiny	Supportive
Unpredictable	Overprotective
Frustrated	Co-dependent

Exhausted	Confused
Inadequate	Tireless
Dependent	Selfless
Searching	A martyr
	Uncomplaining
	Stoical

In that earlier essay I pointed out how nicely some of the stereotypes above fit together like pieces of a puzzle.

Exhausted — Tireless
Restricted — Overprotective
Dependent — Co-dependent

After destroying the "caretaker" and "patient" labels in my own life, I wondered if I needed any labels at all for others and myself. I came up with one. Shortly after banning "caretaker" and "patient" from my vocabulary and mindset, I realized I let other labels such as "writer," "consultant" and "dad" control too much of my life. These labels also supported a host of responsibilities and related stereotypes that boxed me in. I took Alyse on a business trip to Las Vegas in February 1997, when she was 14. Before leaving, I told myself to take off the labels "dad" and "daughter." My view of the label "dad" entails a person who indulges in steady doses of lecturing and worrying. Instead of wearing that label on the trip, I decided that my daughter and I would spend two days being Gregg and Alyse going on an adventure. We had a lot more fun than if we had played out the script of "dad" and "daughter." Sure, I was still her dad and would protect her in any way. But thinking of ourselves as "Gregg and Alyse," instead of the old labels, loosened me up and helped Alyse relax, too.

I still pondered though, whether any labels are necessary to define who I am and who other people are. So I spent a week searching for a label that would be both accurate and freeing in the way I viewed others and myself. After thinking and writing about my search for the perfect label, I finally came up with one I like a whole lot. Here it is.

I am an imperfect man going on a journey of life.

Yes, it's rather long for a label, but it says a whole lot in just 11 words. A saint (and some "caretakers") must try to live up to the impossible standard of perfection. An imperfect person knows he or she will blow it sometimes. In addition, a journey is full of surprises along the way. A journey devoid of mystery and bumps, and even a crisis or two, is not worthy of the word "journey." The unexpected becomes the expected. I no longer have to panic or feel cheated when life treats me a bit rough. That's the nature of journeys. That's life; the ultimate journey.

A day or two after coming up with a suitable label for myself, I realized I could apply the same label to others, loved ones as well as strangers.

She is an imperfect woman going on a journey of life.

I tell myself, yes, Sherrie forgot to be here when our insurance man showed up. But hey, she's got a million things on her mind right now.

He is an imperfect man going on a journey of life.

I tell myself, yes, that guy driving the Corvette just cut in front of me, but I've done the same thing to others when I'm in a hurry.

She is an imperfect girl going on a journey of life.

I tell myself to ease up on Alyse and Corlet, who will and should make mistakes as they journey into young adulthood.

He is an imperfect boy going on a journey of life.

I tell myself that Bret's miscues are helping him – and me – learn important lessons about our separate journeys.

Now, before you get the idea I pretend to be perfect based on my responses above, let me remind you I am an imperfect man on a journey of life. I often respond to situations much differently than what I wrote above. But what I have found is that when I remember the labels, I tend to be more understanding and forgiving in my interactions with others. While I love the fact that every person is unique, my label recognizes that we all have two things in common: 1) we are imperfect and 2) we are all on a complex and difficult journey. A gravestone epitaph in a cemetery in New England reads: "I, too, stranger, was just like you."

Psychologist and author M. Scott Peck wrote, "Life is not a problem to be solved, but a mystery to be lived." When I neglect these labels I have created, I often tend to get bogged down by problems. However, I love the concept of mysteries, which overflow with challenges and struggles and miscues and adventures and intermittent victories. Business guru and author Tom Peters says, "Success is the most boring thing I can think of. Failure is what is interesting and brings growth."

I definitely advise that you delete the "caretaker" and "patient" labels from your life. And I suggest you be careful about trying to live up to confining or negative labels related to other aspects of your life. If you agree with me that some overriding label is appropriate and helpful, come up with your own or borrow mine. Whatever you decide, remember that you are imperfect as you go on your life journey. Revel in the mystery and freedom of that knowledge.

The "X" Factor

— *or* —

Comrades in Arms

A merican men are generally long on material goods and short on friendships. A few years ago I read the results of a study that showed many American men did not have what they considered a trusted friend. When forced to name a best friend, many simply listed the husbands of their wives' best friends. These were men who only occasionally got together as part of a foursome with their wives. They rarely, if ever, spent time alone together playing or conversing at any length. That study partially reveals the shocking and sad state of male friendships in America. It is even more disturbing if you consider a typical male "caretaker" trying to deal with a loved one's chronic illness. Oh yes, such a person might have many friends who are co-workers, but it is unlikely they can talk at a deep level, especially since most companies and work teams operate primarily in the pseudo-community phase.

In lieu of having close friends, "caretakers" could talk to their ill partners. I obviously encourage such couples to communicate "beyond chaos" in phases three and four. On the other hand, "caretakers" might also shell out money to talk to a counselor, which was beneficial for me and could be for others as well. But sometimes, there is nothing like seeking the companionship of those often untapped gems known as friends, who can potentially make this journey alongside chronic illness more bearable.

The "X" factor in sports refers to a key element that could determine the contest's outcome. The "X" factor might be a home-field advantage or the performance of a gifted but erratic young point guard. An "X" factor for those who support chronically ill loved ones might be the presence or absence of one or more buddies. A red warning flag appears in my brain if you tell me you don't have one or more buddies. The absence of friends can decrease your odds of effectively handling the challenge of chronic illness.

I purposely use the term buddies in this essay. Various dictionaries that define "buddy" use words such as comrade, mate and brother. The relationship of true buddies is so natural and free-flowing that it's hard to put into words. Hollywood has done an excellent job in portraying the feel of buddy relationships, though. Some of the best buddy flicks that come to mind are "Butch Cassidy and the Sundance Kid," "Thelma & Louise" and "Return of the Jedi." In each of these movies, buddies rely on each other to get through ordeals. Mere acquaintances and pseudo community friends relate to you on a superficial level, often pretending that life is a piece of cake. Buddies, however, understand that life itself can be an ordeal and they help each other out as comrades in arms.

In August 1997, I took four days off from work and flew to Oregon to visit my buddy John, who lives in a little farmhouse in the countryside not too far from the University of Oregon campus. The old "caretaker" inside me would never have approved of such a visit. It took income out of my family's pocket and took me miles away from the people I must protect. But the wiser person inside me told me that John and I both needed an injection of what I'll call "buddyship." What did two middle-aged men without access to a TV or corporate office do for four days? Well, we attended a minor league baseball game, talked about eternity while looking at a zillion stars in the rural night sky, hit rocks into Dorena Lake in a self-made World Series, talked about the concepts of being versus doing, laughed for long stretches at a time, and went on a magical hike through a forest. John deserves much credit for this book, because he and I have been co-travelers on the journey of self-growth.

We have helped each other along the way, often through the magic of e-mail.

"Ewww," I wrote John a few weeks after my visit, "your last letter bummed me out. Not because you were sad rather than happy, but because you seemed the grim and defeated person of old. Excuse me for being so blunt, but I think we gave each other permission to get on each other's case." John responded to my e-mail message by writing: "Let me give you a piece of my mind – thanks. I needed that. There is no greater sign of sincere friendship than when your bud slaps you on the helmet to wake you up. And everything you said was right on. I kept your e-mail and will read it often, because I do feel grim, though with friends like you, not defeated." Good buddies are oft-neglected shields against total defeat by life's challenges, including chronic illness.

Greg has been a good bud since the summer after our senior year of high school. We were inseparable for several years. Now we both find ourselves in middle age with wives, kids and mortgages. We are like brothers to each other and are not afraid to say so. We don't see each other much anymore, but when we do, it's as if we were apart for only a few days. Last week Greg called me long distance "just so I could laugh," he said. Greg and I do not limit our relationship to yuks, though. We call upon each other whenever our spouses or parents are ill, we seek each other's advice on our separate careers, and we talk about our fears and frustrations. Buddies may seek each other out to share a few laughs, but they are just as open to sharing tears.

Kyle and I were boyhood chums. When Kyle moved to Montana, during our sophomore year of high school, it marked the end of our frequent times together. Now, we see each other about once a decade and call or write about twice a year. Minutes after Greg and I had finished talking to each other on the telephone one day, I called Kyle. We talked about our old baseball card games, about the Mariners and Rockies, about our respective kids.

"And how is your lovely wife Sherrie?" he said in jovial voice.

"Oh, Kyle," I said, "she's really struggling. Her damn hips are still screwed up from the truck accident."

"Oh man, I'm sorry to hear that," he said in a solemn voice. "And here I've been worried about my little problems all day. How are you doing? I feel so badly for you, Gregg. Man, let's each hop in our cars and meet in Bozeman for a beer." I truly believe if I had said I would meet him there in 12 hours he would have headed for Bozeman. We talked a bit more about Sherrie and other things and then I said I had to get going. Just before we hung up, my tough Montana friend said, "I love you, Gregg. Hang in there."

Who knows, it might be a felony in Montana to tell a male friend "I love you." I'll tell you what, though. It becomes much easier to "hang in there" with buddies such as John, Greg and Kyle (and Andy, Steve and Wild Bill). By the way, I consider my buddies and myself to be relatively strong guys. You would want us on your side in a street fight. Even more impressive than our physical prowess, though, is our courage to be vulnerable; perhaps that's our major strength as men. If you are without a buddy, make it a priority to find one. Seek out people with common interests and then, over time, break out of the pseudo-community phase. Be willing to "dig down deep" as you share your thoughts and feelings. Ask open-ended questions to help your would-be buddy open up more.

My buddies and I never have to hide out together as a contemporary "Hole in the Wall Gang" or fight Darth Vader and the forces of evil. But we have stood and will continue to stand together as comrades in the battles of life.

Baby-Boomer Blues

— or —

Careers & the Spirit

Society expects a "caretaker" to be a saint and a martyr. We are never supposed to complain while making sacrifices for others, especially the "patient." So you can imagine the bafflement of some people when I seriously considered leaving a secure and decent job as public relations manager for a Fortune 100 company. A lot of people considered me crazy. Though they didn't say it aloud, some labeled me selfish.

But here's the deal. I was dying a slow death in a large corporation. Some people would relish being a part of the huge machine that is a Fortune 100 company. Others, me included, like to ride the career range in smaller groups or as "Lone Rangers." As you already know, chronic illness creates loss in a family and among individuals. You might lose financial freedom and time with friends and options for recreation, among other things. I felt as if my family was in a holding pattern of survival. I seemed to be in a similar kind of holding pattern at work. I was unable to take chances, so I felt my real skills were being wasted. Get the picture? I felt stifled at home and at work, which covers just about all the bases. Maybe it is because I grew up in those heady post-World War II days, when America and freedom danced together in the spotlight of a global ballroom. I nearly go crazy spending 10 minutes going through customs at a Mexican airport. I hate being told I can't do something. The subtle and not-so-subtle messages baby boomers received daily as kids were that our options were countless and the only real barriers were our collective inability or unwillingness to go for the gold. We were free to become whatever we wanted to be.

Those people who came of age in the 1960s also sought idealistic goals. Unfortunately, my public relations goals seemed meaningless and I felt I had the freedom of your average zoo tiger. The messages we baby boomers heard proved to be somewhat incorrect. However, I still feel their spirit flowing through my veins, and truth be known, feel thankful for those messages that hailed the glory of freedom and idealism. I suppose that makes me a true-blue baby boomer. But for much of the 1980s, I felt boxed in. I was the mime who discovers glass surrounds him on all sides. Sherrie and I let chronic illness construct an invisible cell around our family and I allowed my mind to consider my job a benign prison.

"Piburn the Prisoner" became "Gregg the Grouch," and "Dad the Depressed," and "Hubby the Hateful." The last thing any family needs is a hateful and depressed grouch for a husband and father. So with a clear conscience I chose to seek other career options, hoping that by finding greater job satisfaction I would also provide greater love and support for my wife and children. My career transition did not come overnight or without hours of consideration. I had always wanted to be my own boss, but thought of taking a calculated risk rather than a leap into a dark abyss. Fortunately, I was able to take advantage of a voluntary severance program offered by my company that gave me a bonus equal to 11 months' salary. Before leaving my position in the corporate world, I lined up a part-time consulting job at the same rate of pay I had been making full-time. Those two safety nets enabled me to break free of the "golden handcuffs" clamped around my wrist by my corporate job and embark on my Lone Ranger career. When I signed on the dotted line that made my departure official, it seemed as if a switch flicked on in my mind. For the first time in years, I felt excited about my career. That excitement spilled over into my personal life as well. Of course the danger of self-employment is that the business can become all-consuming. Soon after I started my consulting business, I developed a personalized career credo, which captures the essence of why I work.

I want a career that enhances the quality of my life.

This credo says my career serves my life. I know people whose lives serve their careers. Remember, I'm an imperfect man on a journey of life, so I sometimes screw up and let my job take precedence over family matters. Even though I don't work at an office 50 or 60 hours weekly anymore, I sometimes think too much about work when I'm at home, but I'm doing that less and less.

My credo has helped me make key life decisions. For example, in 1994 I started a long and complex application process to become a part-time trainer for an international training organization. The arrangement was that I would still run my own company, but gain national exposure as a trainer, speaker and consultant. I told the execs at the training organization that I had to limit my travel days to five per month, which I thought my family and I could handle. After my first four out-of-town trips, I realized it was not working. However, I remembered all the hoops the company and I jumped through to create this business relationship. I thought about how well I had done in the training sessions. Bowing out after such a short stint would embarrass me. Then my credo flashed onto my mental screen.

I want a career that enhances the quality of my life.

OK, Piburn, is this training gig enhancing or harming the quality of your life? The answer came quickly. This much travel is harmful for everyone in the family. I met with the company's recruiter and training manager. I shocked them by saying I intended to end the business relationship. I reminded them of my family situation, especially Sherrie's chronic illness. Then I told them my credo. They were impressed someone actually had developed a credo and were even more shocked I chose to live by it. "We can't argue with that," the recruiter said. "We're sorry you're leaving, but glad you're doing it for the right reasons."

As I grow older I'm more aware of the challenge of finding the fine line of a balanced life. I crossed that line by thinking I could travel five days per month. But I would be crossing the line on the other side if I caved in to the pressure of becoming a corporate employee again. The fine line for my business seems to include finding regional clients and limiting out-of-state work opportunities. When I do fly to a distant job, I often take one of our children with me. I now focus more on writing, which can provide me broader recognition from the comfort of my home office.

I love to write, speak to groups, facilitate retreats and train and coach executives, and I've found a way to do all of those things within the boundaries of my credo and my family's needs. In 1972, Studs Terkel published a book titled, *Working*. In it, the Chicago writer had interviewed hundreds of Americans about their jobs. Nora Watson, an organizational communicator, told Terkel: "Most of us have jobs that are too small for our spirits. Our real imaginations have not yet been challenged." During the first few years of Sherrie's illness, my job was too small for my spirit. And my frustrated spirit was too small to come alive to better love and support Sherrie. The challenge of having a successful career and family life is to work out a way in which you can create a career that enlivens your spirit, while at the same time, love and support the most important people in your life. I did it and so can you.

Lightening the Load

— *or* —

Strengthening the Wolf

For many people, getting Christmas tree lights out of storage and putting them up is an exciting annual event. In the late 1970s and early 1980s, an exciting annual event for me was getting our cross-country skis out of storage and attaching the ski rack to our car. Sherrie and I were young, healthy – and poor. Although we both loved to downhill ski, the cost and time involved made it a rare event for us. But living along the front range of the Rockies placed us within 45 minutes of wonderful cross-country ski terrain. We would often join a group of exuberant friends for an afternoon of slicing through the snow on tree-lined trails. Other times, Sherrie and I would finish Sunday lunch and agree to head up to the canyon and ski for a couple of hours by ourselves. We dodged lift lines and trail fees.

I loved to follow Sherrie up the trails as her strong legs powered her through the snow, sometimes for 20-minute stretches without rest. We were both teaching aerobics classes back then and Sherrie also conducted cross-country ski lessons once or twice during the week. We were in great shape and used our physical fitness to power our recreational and entertainment pursuits. When we went out to ski, we would occasionally see an older couple on skinny skis, going at a slow but steady pace up and down the trails. Gray hair rimmed their heads and they wore smiles on their tanned faces. Without talking about it, Sherrie and I viewed these older skiers as visions of our future – always staying fit, always living near the mountains, always having the skis handy, always ready for some excitement or peace on the mountain trails of winter.

The avalanche of chronic illness crushed that vision. Once Sherrie's symptoms kicked in, she was as capable of spending an afternoon on skinny skis as I would have been swimming the English Channel. The closest we came to skiing for several years was watching the Winter Olympics on TV. Her skis – and mine – stayed in storage year after year. I started to get soft around the gut and mad around my heart. But, in my quest to be the perfect "caretaker," I kept a stiff upper lip while refraining from doing what I loved to do – strapping on the skis. Guilt prevented me from driving into the Rocky Mountains with only my skis on the rack.

I had stuffed Sherrie's chronic illness into an imaginary backpack and hoisted it onto my shoulders. I wanted her illness to be as big a burden on me as it was on her. I thought – in my co-dependent mind – that I was doing Sherrie a favor by making myself suffer with her. Instead, I was hurting Sherrie, my kids and myself.

By putting in storage a part of myself that gave me joy and peace, I was creating a frustrated, miserable and angry man of myself. Oh yeah, that's being supportive to my family, isn't it? It was as if my actions and emotions were saying: "I'm home, doing my duties, not having any fun, being the perfect husband, father and 'caretaker.' Now, while I'm here with all of you – rather than up in the mountains – let me spread a healthy dose of frustration, misery and anger throughout the household." Unbelievably, I thought I was doing the perfect thing based on the circumstances. I felt like a pouting little boy who could no longer play football because his friend took the ball home with him.

Yes, I needed to help support Sherrie and my children. But loving and effective support do not come clothed in frustration, misery and anger. To love others, you must love yourself. Likewise, to support others, you have to support yourself. I finally realized that supporting myself meant finding time to do what I'm good at and what gives me pleasure. Rudyard Kipling wrote, "The strength of the pack is the wolf and the strength of the wolf is the pack." One way to help my pack was to become stronger myself, not busier fulfilling "caretaker" duties, but stronger building my physical, mental, emotional and spiritual health.

As I started to grieve the loss of the healthy Sherrie, I started being more honest with her and a few good buddies. They all encouraged me to take better care of myself. Sherrie is the person who most often tells me to take a break, call a friend, pack up my skis and head for the hills. I know she wishes she could go . . . and I have not given up hope that one day she will. But for now, she feels less guilt about her illness, knowing that I occasionally do physical activities that invigorate me. And she knows that I will come home without the frustration, misery and anger that used to dwell inside me day after day. I don't go skiing as much as I did early on in our marriage, but the skis are out of storage and my attitude is better than it was a few years ago. That mythical backpack I carry is lighter now . . . and so is my heart.

SECTION FOUR ACTION PAGE

Without Action, It's Only Words

1. List the elements of your "voice"

What are some of the aspects that make up your voice? Remember, they might relate to your philosophies, skills, interests or attitudes. List four or five elements of your voice.

a. _____

b. _____

c. _____

d _____

e. _____

Now, go back to the elements you listed above. In the right margin write the word (or letter) high (h), medium (m) or low (l) next to each one to rate the degree to which each element is being expressed in your life. For example, if you listed "creativity" as an element and believe you have many opportunities to let that part of yourself shine, then put an "h" at the end of that line. However, if you listed "humorous" as an element, but feel that your humor is being stifled, put an "l" next to that line. If you have an "h" next to all your elements, then you are a fortunate man or woman. If you have one or more "l's," try to determine ways to let those elements shine more in your life.

2. Develop an honest and healthy label

In recent years I have tried to eliminate labels from my vocabulary and mindset. I definitely have tried to slay the labels "caretaker" and "patient." Perhaps you will also decide, as I did, that it benefits you to apply a different kind of label to others and yourself. As a reminder, what I came up with was: "I am an imperfect man on a journey of life" or "He/she is an imperfect man/woman on a journey of life." Develop your own labels and write a brief paragraph in your notebook explaining how living by these labels could have a positive impact on your interactions with others and boost your self-esteem.

Label for me: _____

Label for others: _____

3. Create a career credo

Remember, a credo is a statement of belief. Keeping that in mind, answer the following questions to help you develop a career credo, which can be an aid in helping you deal with the impact of chronic illness.

• What tangible rewards do you seek from work?

_____
_____
_____

• What intangible rewards do you seek from work?

_____

_____

_____

• What do those closest to you need from your work?

_____

_____

_____

• Now put it all together and write one statement that represents your career credo. You know you have a good one if it influences your behavior and helps you make critical decisions.

_____

_____

_____

4. Mine for gold

• Out of all the essays and suggested activities in this chapter, what do you believe is the most significant and/or memorable nugget for you?

_____

_____

_____

• What is the first step you will take toward making that nugget truly impact your life for the better?

• I will _____ (what?)
by _____ (when?)
EXAMPLE: I will describe my fears about my significant other's upcoming operation by the end of the week.

note

In the Section One Action Page, I asked readers to consider how, if at all, they were treating an ill loved one like a "china doll." I asked readers to discuss this topic with their loved one AFTER reading the entire book. If a china-doll issue exists, talk about it openly and honestly in the next day or two.

A FEW FINAL THOUGHTS

(Thanks for reading the book. Sherrie
and I hope it will help you meet
the challenges of living with
chronic illness together.)

Hard Lessons

— *or* —

Wise Kids

If you have three or more children, you know it is hard for them to agree on anything. But on at least one topic, my three children agree: Living with chronic illness has been hard. They have seen Sherrie and me get angry over minor issues because of the stress of dealing with chronic illness and other difficulties. They have missed out on some activities because of Sherrie's health problems. However, they also have learned some important lessons.

"I've learned not to give up," says Alyse. "I need to take life one day at a time."

Corlet says: "I've learned that life doesn't always go the way you think it will."

Bret has learned something about pitching in and taking responsibility. "Come on, let's get the rowboat out ourselves. Mom's back hurts, so she can't help."

What advice would my children give to other families battling chronic illness? BE OPEN AND HONEST ABOUT THE ILLNESS. In other words, "turn on the lights" instead of keeping your children in the dark. At the same time, I believe it's important not to frequently refer to chronic illness as the family's villain in front of the kids because it tends to make the person who is sick a semi-villain. This is a lesson I learned while journeying through the four phases. It's also unwise to repeatedly praise your ill loved one for her courage and perseverance in front of the children. It might come across as phony, like a bad public-relations program. Over time the children will see, through the ill person's actions, just how courageous he or she is. "Turn on the lights" and let your children pick up on the valuable lessons in their own time.

Great Reading

— *or* —

"Turn on the Lights"

My Favorites

Personal Growth

Buechner, Frederick. *Telling Secrets: A Memoir.* New York: HarperCollins Publishers, 1991.

Hansel, Tim. *You Gotta Keep Dancin': In the Midst of Life's Hurts, You Can Choose Joy!* Colorado Springs, CO: Chariot Victor, 1998

James, John, and Frank Cherry. *The Grief Recovery Handbook: A Step-by-Step Program for Moving Beyond Loss.* New York: Harper & Row Publishers, 1988.

Jones, Alan. *Soul Making: The Desert Way of Spirituality.* New York: HarperCollins Publishers, 1985.

Mason, Mike. *The Mystery of Marriage: As Iron Sharpens Iron.* Portland, OR: Multnomah Press, 1985.

Peck, M. Scott, MD. *The Road Less Traveled: A New Psychology of Love, Traditional Values and Spiritual Growth.* Second Edition. New York: Simon & Schuster, 1998.

Peck, M. Scott, MD. *A World Waiting to be Born: Civility Rediscovered.* New York: Bantam Books, 1993.

Sheehy, Gail. *New Passages: Mapping Your Life Across Time.* New York: Random House, 1995.

Career Growth

Csikszentmihalyi, Mihaly. *Flow: The Psychology of Optimal Experience.* New York: Harper & Row Publishers, 1990.

Goleman, Daniel. *Emotional Intelligence: Why it Can Matter More than IQ.* New York: Bantam Books, 1995.

Whyte, David. *The Heart Aroused: Poetry and Preservation of the Soul.* New York: Doubleday, 1994.

Whyte, David. *The Heart Aroused: Poetry and the Preservation of the Soul in Corporate America.* New York: Doubleday, 1994.

Fiction

Greene, Graham. *The Power and the Glory.* New York: Penguin Classics, 1991.

Hugo, Victor. *Les Miserables.* New York: Viking Penguin, 1997 (reissue date).

Saroyan, William. *The Human Comedy.* New York: Dell Publishing, 1943.

Steinbeck, John. *The Grapes of Wrath.* New York: Penguin Books, 1939.

Available from the Arthritis Foundation (800/207-8633)

Books

Arthritis Foundation. *250 Tips for Making Life with Arthritis Easier.* Marietta, GA: Longstreet Press, 1997.

Arthritis Foundation. *Arthritis 101: Questions You Have. Answers You Need.* Marietta, GA: Longstreet Press, 1997.

Arthritis Foundation. *Health Organizer: A Personal Health-Care Record.* Atlanta: Arthritis Foundation, 1998.

Arthritis Foundation. *Primer on the Rheumatic Diseases.* Edition 11. Atlanta, Arthritis Foundation, 1997.

Arthritis Foundation. *Raising a Child with Arthritis: A Parent's Guide.* Atlanta: Arthritis Foundation, 1998.

Arthritis Foundation. *Toward Healthy Living: A Wellness Journal.* Atlanta: Arthritis Foundation, 1998.

Arthritis Foundation. *Your Personal Guide to Living Well with Fibromyalgia.* Marietta, GA: Longstreet Press, 1997.

Periodicals

Arthritis Today. Bimonthly magazine for Arthritis Foundation members.

Bulletin on the Rheumatic Diseases. Monthly newsletter for health-care professionals.

Fibromyalgia Wellness Letter. Bimonthly newsletter for people with fibromyalgia.

Kids Get Arthritis Too: A Wellness Letter. Bimonthly newsletter for American Juvenile Arthritis Organization participants.

Videotapes

Fibromyalgia Interval Training. A warm-water exercise program.

Pathways to Better Living with Arthritis. An exercise program for those with limited mobility.

PACE (People with Arthritis Can Exercise) I & II. Land exercise programs.

PEP (Pool Exercise Program). An aquatic exercise program.

Seven Summary Themes

— or —

In Case You Missed Them

Itried to focus this book on a few key themes. Just in case you missed them, here are some of the themes I think are most important.

1. Life is difficult.

Don't deny that truth or freeze up because of it. Take on each challenge – including "The Intruder" – as it comes.

2. Rid yourself of confining labels.

Delete from your vocabulary and your behavior the labels "caretaker" and "patient." Chronic illness thrives on patsies who live by those insidious and wicked labels.

3. Turn on the lights.

Problems such as chronic illness often force people to freeze up or hide their emotions in the dark. Illuminate your life through open, honest and courageous communication conducted "above the barbed wire."

4. Tap into "The Fat Lady."

Despite the horrid nature of chronic illness, it provides lessons about yourself, your loved one and life. Chronic illness has taken plenty from you, so take some life lessons from it.

5. Take care of yourself.

The last thing your loved one needs is a friend/lover/ spouse/child who is also physically, mentally or emotionally wounded. By taking care of your own health, you will be better able to truly and lovingly support your ill loved one.

6. Swallow your pride.

Don't try to go through this alone. Tap into support groups, accept offers of help, pay for house cleaners and counselors (if possible), and rely on some buddies.

7. Fight back!

You fight back against "The Intruder" by making and sticking to commitments, by breaking out of the pseudo-community and chaos phases, by "turning on the lights" with medical professionals and loved ones, by regaining as much control as possible, by letting your actions scream, "Freeeeeeeeedommmmmmmm!"

Hope Dies Last

— *or* —

Freeeeeeeedommmmmmm!

A summer ago, I watched Sherrie wince as the specialist jabbed a long needle into her back. As the doctor twisted and shoved the needle even farther into my wife's body, she inhaled deeply, then slowly exhaled. I held her hand and thought how easy it would be for Sherrie to decline this procedure. Yet, she was willing to choose discomfort then, in hopes of decreasing pain later. Unless you are a police officer or firefighter, most people don't have to show courage on a regular basis. My wife does and for that I think she is courageous.

Once when Sherrie was serving as my personal editor for this book, she stated that something I had written about her upset her greatly. She "turned on a light" by confronting me about it, which I thought was another courageous act. I confess I took a quick trip to the outskirts of pseudo-community, trying briefly to downplay her anger. But before making myself at home "beneath the barbed wire," I heard Sherrie say how my response belittled her thoughts and feelings about the matter in question. I quickly thought through the options, including the one of choosing discomfort over comfort. We heard each other out, validated each other's feelings, and eventually came to common ground. Through the discomfort of disagreement, we came away with a stronger relationship.

These relatively simple anecdotes reveal how two people can fight back against "The Intruder." They represent ways in which we seek to maintain control of our lives, while also seeking personal growth, and a stronger bond between us. In the introduction to this book, I said there would be no fairy-tale endings. Sherrie continues to battle fibromyalgia, migraine headaches and pain in her back and hips, but her mind and spirit have grown stronger over the years. I continue to make mistakes, but find myself above "the barbed wire" more often than below it. There's a Spanish saying that goes like this: *La esperanza muere al ultimo.* It means, "Hope dies last." I hope that message of hope comes through in these pages.

In the Oscar-winning movie "Braveheart," protagonist William Wallace, portrayed by Mel Gibson, leads a Scottish rebellion against an evil British king (symbolic of "The Intruder") and his minions. Wallace and his comrades also contend with certain Scottish clans, whose leaders become accomplices to the king. Ultimately, the bad guys capture Wallace, but not before he has weakened them with his moxie, perseverance and leadership. Wallace's last word, screamed with passion just before the executioner finishes his deadly task, is "Freeeeeeeeedommmmmmm!" His message and leadership lived on beyond his death.

I could meekly and silently let "The Intruder" and its accomplices destroy Sherrie and my family at will. Instead, I view my writing this book as one way to fight back against chronic illness, verbal fists punching as I scream, "Freeeeeeeee-dommmmmmmm!" Perhaps my message will live on through this book. So I encourage, no, I challenge you and your loved one to fight back against chronic illness. The fight makes you stronger as individuals, couples, families. That new, stronger bond becomes a powerful, upgraded weapon in the ongoing war. Let the enemy and the listening world hear your cry of "Freeeeeeeeedommmmmmmm!"

— *Gregg Piburn*

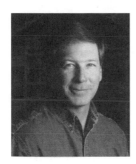

About the Author

GREGG PIBURN

"As the world grows more complex, the need for simple, face-to-face communication is heightened."

Gregg Piburn is the President and owner of Leader's Edge Consulting, Inc., where he advises and trains managers and their teams to be more courageous, effective and satisfied through better communication. He uses these same elements when working as a public speaker at conferences across the country.

Raised in Colorado, Piburn earned his BA in Journalism from Colorado State University and worked as a newspaper columnist, reporter and editor, winning several awards. He then went on to work for a Fortune 100 company as a communications manager. He has also worked for many years as a freelance writer and has been published in a variety of corporate, sports and health magazines.

In addition to the responsibilities of his job, he and his wife Sherrie give half-day workshops for people impacted by chronic illness.

Above all, Piburn is devoted to his family. He and Sherrie have three children: Corlet, Alyse and Bret. He spends his free time helping coach his son's sports teams, cross-country and downhill skiing, riding his motorcycle, reading and exercising. If Piburn isn't at home or at work, he and his family are probably enjoying their rustic cabin in the Rockies.

OTHER GREAT BOOKS
ARTHRITIS FOUNDATION® from the Arthritis Foundation

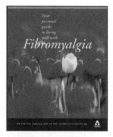

Your Guide to Living Well with Fibromyalgia
This hands-on workbook gives you the tools to get control over your condition and take the first steps toward wellness.
224 pages, #835–203
$14.95

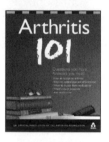

Arthritis 101: Questions You Have. Answers You Need.
Get the fundamental text that gives you concise, easy-to-understand answers to even your most basic questions.
144 pages, #835–201
$11.95

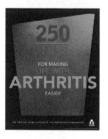

250 Tips for Making Life With Arthritis Easier
Packed with simple ideas for making your daily tasks easier on your joints and less fatiguing, this book gives you ideas that you can start using today!
88 pages, #835–202
$9.95

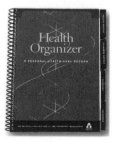

Health Organizer: A Personal Health–Care Record
Keep your medical and insurance records in one easy-to-find location, and track your symptoms with useful prompts in this spiral-bound, tabbed organizer.
144 pages, #835–207
$14.95

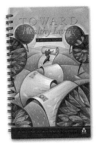

Toward Healthy Living: A Wellness Journal

This beautifully designed, spiral-bound journal contains inspirational quotes and pain and mood charts that help you track the progress of your health.

144 pages, #835-205
$14.95

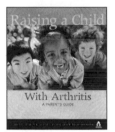

Raising a Child With Arthritis: A Parent's Guide

This essential guide to understanding and coping with the challenges of childhood arthritis gives you reliable advice and information from top pediatric health professionals.

194 pages, #835-209
$14.95

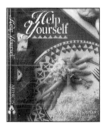

Help Yourself: Recipes and Resources from the Arthritis Foundation

This limited-edition cookbook contains nearly 250 healthy and easy-to-prepare recipes as well as information on special devices that simplify food preparation.

158 pages, #835-204
ONLY $12.95

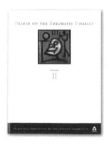

Primer on the Rheumatic Diseases

This highly technical text was originally written for medical professionals and contains the latest information on the science, diagnosis and treatments for most rheumatic conditions.

516 pages, #750-3250
$39.95

See Next Page for Ordering Information

Order Arthritis Foundation Books Today

using one of three easy methods:

PHONE:
1–800–207–8633
Operators are available to take your
order Monday – Friday, 8 a.m. – 6 p.m. EST

MAIL:
Send order form and payment (credit card, check or money order) **to:**
Arthritis Foundation Distribution Center
P.O. Box 1616
Alpharetta, GA 30009–1616

FAX:
770–442–9742 (credit card orders only)

ITEM #	TITLE	QTY.	PRICE	TOTAL

*SHIPPING & HANDLING:		

Inside the U.S. .... Up to $25.00 add $4.99
.... 25.01 to $60.00 add $5.99
.... Over $60.00 add 10% of order
Outside the U.S. (Air Mail Only) add 40% of order
If you require priority shipping (second day), add $20 to
the charge marked on the chart.

Subtotal	$
*Shipping	$
Total	$

Please allow up to two weeks for ground domestic delivery. Return of items in salable condition
are accepted within 30 days of shipping date. Shipping and handling will not be refunded.

METHOD OF PAYMENT (choose one)

O Check or money order enclosed

O Purchase order enclosed ($200 minimum for purchase orders)

O VISA* O MasterCard* O American Express* *($10 minimum)

SIGNATURE _____

TELEPHONE # _____ EXP. DATE _____

CREDIT CARD NUMBER ⬚⬚⬚⬚ ⬚⬚⬚⬚ ⬚⬚⬚⬚ ⬚⬚⬚⬚

BILL TO: Name _____

Organization _____

Address _____

City _____

State/Zip _____

Phone _____ AF Member # _____

SHIP TO: Name _____

Organization _____

Address _____

City _____

State/Zip _____

Phone _____ AF Member # _____

PAYMENT:
We accept check, money order or credit card (VISA, MasterCard, American Express) payments. There is a minimum purchase of $10 when using a credit card. Please note that all checks and money orders must be in U.S. dollars drawn on a U.S. bank and made out to the Arthritis Foundation.

PURCHASE ORDERS:
Purchase orders will be accepted for institutional orders exceeding $200. Please include a copy of the authorized purchase order with your materials order form. The Arthritis Foundation reserves the right to deny any purchase order or require prepayment.

RETURNS:
Returns of items in salable condition are accepted within 30 days of shipping date. Shipping and handling will not be refunded. Please call 800-207-8633 if you are not satisfied with your order or want to return it.

SOURCE CODE: PIBURN